THETAHEALING™

THETA HEALING™

Introducing an
Extraordinary Energy
Healing Modality

Vianna Stibal

HAY HOUSE

Carlsbad, California • New York City • London
Sydney •Johannesburg • Vancouver • New Delhi

First published and distributed in the United Kingdom by:
Hay House UK Ltd, Astley House, 33 Notting Hill Gate, London W11 3JQ
Tel: +44 (0)20 3675 2450; Fax: +44 (0)20 3675 2451; www.hayhouse.co.uk

Published and distributed in the United States of America by:
Hay House Inc., PO Box 5100, Carlsbad, CA 92018-5100
Tel: (1) 760 431 7695 or (800) 654 5126
Fax: (1) 760 431 6948 or (800) 650 5115; www.hayhouse.com

Published and distributed in Australia by:
Hay House Australia Ltd, 18/36 Ralph St, Alexandria NSW 2015
Tel: (61) 2 9669 4299; Fax: (61) 2 9669 4144; www.hayhouse.com.au

Published and distributed in the Republic of South Africa by:
Hay House SA (Pty) Ltd, PO Box 990, Witkoppen 2068
info@hayhouse.co.za; www.hayhouse.co.za

Published and distributed in India by:
Hay House Publishers India, Muskaan Complex, Plot No.3, B-2,
Vasant Kunj, New Delhi 110 070
Tel: (91) 11 4176 1620; Fax: (91) 11 4176 1630; www.hayhouse.co.in

Distributed in Canada by:
Raincoast Books, 2440 Viking Way, Richmond, B.C. V6V 1N2
Tel: (1) 604 448 7100; Fax: (1) 604 270 7161; www.raincoast.com

A catalogue record for this book is available from the British Library.

ISBN: 978-1-84850-243-7

Previously published by Rolling Thunder Publishing, Idaho, ISBN 978-0-9671754-2-3
Printed and bound by CPI Group (UK) Ltd, Croydon, CR0 4YY

This book is dedicated:

To my God, the Creator of All That Is. It was under divine direction that the information contained in this book was received.

To my mother, who taught me to pray and to believe that God always hears and answers our prayers.

To my husband, who compiled the writing for this book, and who assisted me during my travels as I taught these techniques to the world. He is appreciated so much more than I could ever express.

To my children, who inspire me, who are my friends and who are all gifted intuitives.

To my precious grandchildren, who have brought blessings and joy into my life.

To all the ThetaHealing instructors and practitioners and the magnificent people throughout the world who have brought it to life. These wonderful people have been a source of joy to me. They are an inspiration to me on my journeys as I present these important techniques and concepts to the world.

And to those I have yet to meet, may your paths lead you to the place of greatest peace and abundant goodness.

Believe nothing,
No matter where you read it,
Or who has said it,
Not even if I have said it,
Unless it agrees with your own reason,
And your common sense.

Buddha

Contents

PREFACE

In this book I will reveal one of the most powerful energy-healing techniques that has ever been written down: ThetaHealing.™ ThetaHealing is a meditational process that brings about physical, psychological and spiritual healing with focused prayer through the Creator. The Creator has freely given us the fascinating knowledge you are about to receive. It has changed my life and the lives of many others.

There is one requirement that is absolute with this technique: you must have a central belief in the Creator of All That Is. I realize that the Creator has many different names, and God, Buddha, Shiva, Goddess, Jesus, Yahweh and Allah are all currents leading in a flow towards the Seventh Plane of Existence and the Creative Energy of All That Is. ThetaHealing has no religious affiliation. Neither are its processes specific to any age, sex, race, colour, creed or religion. Anyone with a pure belief in God or the Creative Force can access and use the branches of the ThetaHealing tree.

This book is a fusion of the past works of *Go Up and Seek God, Go Up and Work with God* and *The DNA 2 Advanced Manual*, with additional information developed since these works were written.

Even though I am sharing this information with you, I do not accept any responsibility for the changes that can occur from its use. The responsibility is yours, a responsibility you assume when you realize that you have the power to change your life as well as the lives of others through permission.

Please note, the remedies, approaches and techniques described herein are not meant to supplement, or be a substitute for, professional medical care or treatment. You should not treat a serious medical ailment without prior consultation from a qualified healthcare professional.

Acknowledgements

A special thanks to Sky A'Hearn for her dedication in all the typing she has done in ThetaHealing classes over the years.

1

THE FORMATION OF THETAHEALING™

From the conception of the Orian Technique in 1994 to what ThetaHealing™ has become in the present day has been quite a journey. This journey has been shared with the wonderful ThetaHealing practitioners and instructors who support the work. ThetaHealing continues to grow as a beautiful tree in spring, watered by the interest of people around the world.

❖❖❖❖❖

My name is Vianna. I am the founder of what has become ThetaHealing. I was born with an inherent intuitive ability, although it was not my original plan to use this ability for healing. I began an initial study of Taoism, nutrition and herbs because of personal health problems. These interests eventually led me along the path to Nature's Path, which is the name of my business.

This path originally began in 1990, when I divorced my husband of 10 years and had three young children to raise. I had heard that the government was required to hire a certain number of women for the Department of Energy. There was a Department of Energy facility relatively close to where I lived in Idaho Falls, Idaho. My plan was to work at what was called the 'Site' in nuclear security and still pursue my true interest in art. I knew that the bus ride to work would be long, but I thought the pay and benefits would be worth the effort.

It was in 1991 that I began the year-long training for the job of nuclear security guard. Competition was fierce and I had to learn skills that pushed me to the limit. After completing my training I took a job at a nearby manufacturing plant while I waited for my security clearance to work for the government.

During this time I never forgot my other interests. On breaks I would draw sketches of the other employees and give them short intuitive readings. This was shift work and I would often work from midnight to morning.

As a single mother, I soon realized that working as a security guard at a manufacturing plant did not offer the future that I wanted for my family. I knew that something had to change.

Health problems provided the incentive I needed to concentrate on the study of naturopathic medicine. Once I had finished the course in naturopathic medicine, in March 1994 I opened a business offering full-time massage, nutritional counselling and a naturopathic practice.

I came to the realization that I was following my life's path when doors began to open. I met a psychic who suggested that I do readings for income. As if by magic I had an office to work in, and from the very first day I always had clients to see. Within the first week I had met the person who was to become my best friend and had established repeat clients for readings. It was during these readings that I found that if I would listen, the voice of the Creator would give me instructions. I became quite good at the readings and was asked to do classes on the technique I was using. This was my beginning as a medical intuitive. From this time forward my metaphysical experiences increased exponentially to quantify who I was to become.

Meanwhile I had developed a severe problem with my right leg. It would intermittently swell up to twice its normal size. Due to the inflammation and severe pain, I decided it was wise to seek conventional medical help. In the August of 1995, I was diagnosed with bone cancer. I was told that I had a tumour in my right femur. Every test that was performed at this time confirmed it. The bone specialist told me that he had seen only two other cases like mine. He also informed me that he felt amputation might be my best option. This, he said, would give me a little more time to live.

I felt as though darkness was gathering about me, and my ordeal was not over yet. My doctor sent me to the University of Utah for a biopsy. I was told that the procedure required my leg to be opened to allow the doctor to go in and take a bone sample by scraping the inside of my femur. I had no choice but to travel for four hours, in excruciating pain, for this biopsy. Blake, my husband at the time, drove me to Utah and I was admitted to hospital. It was necessary for me to be awake for the procedure, forced to listen to the sounds of the hammer and drill. I was advised to stay in hospital overnight, but Blake told the hospital staff that we were leaving because we had no insurance. I was too weak to argue with him. So, in incredible pain, I was bustled to the car and taken to spend the night at Blake's brother's house before the long drive home.

As I was leaving hospital, I was told by the doctors that if I walked on my leg it would break. If this happened there would be no alternative but to amputate it to prevent the spread of the cancer. I was also informed that I might only have a couple of months to live anyway.

This ordeal put me on crutches for six weeks. I was still in unbearable pain from the tumour. My life seemed to be falling apart. I hobbled around on the crutches, living with constant pain and doubt as to how much longer I could actually survive. Still I went forward, continuing to see clients, not because of great courage or endurance, but because I had financial obligations and my young children needed me. Even though I was newly married to Blake, the relationship was anything but a true partnership and was an added burden on my declining health. I couldn't just give up and die, leaving my children alone. The very thought of them being sent to relatives, even to their father (who was paraplegic and ill), was unbearable. These thoughts gave me the will to live.

Even though I was very ill, my intuitive abilities became even more accurate, as did my connection to the Creator. All my life I had believed that I had a higher purpose from a promise that I made when I was 17. Now I was uncertain if I would complete it.

In confusion and sadness I sent forth a cry to the Creator: 'Why me? Why am I losing my leg? God, am I going to die? I have so much left to do!'

In the middle of this plea I heard a voice, as loud and clear as if the speaker was standing right next to me in the room: 'Vianna, you are here with or without a leg, so deal with it.'

I was astonished by this answer, but, although I didn't know it at the time, it was just what I needed. In that instant I became even more determined to find a way to heal my body.

Healers from the area where I lived heard of my plight and people came from seemingly everywhere to help me. Some were wonderful healers, which I am sure kept me going through the dark times. The prayers that were made on my behalf kept me alive. I still thank God for Alice and Barbara helping to take away the pain.

I was a pitiful sight, hobbling into my office, leaning on my massage table to do massages and painfully struggling through readings. Adding to my problems, I had developed a staph infection in my leg. I decided that *enough was enough!* I was going to treat myself.

First, let me say that I have never been against conventional medicine. I believe that we should respect the opinions of trained healthcare professionals and in most cases they are likely to be correct. Even so, I felt that in my isolated case the doctors were wrong in their diagnosis of bone cancer.

I trusted my intuition and the information I was receiving from the Creator and I began putting my knowledge of naturopathy to good use. I realized that it was vital for me to focus on aggressively cleaning out my body. I began a series of lemon cleanses as well as sauna cleanses. I spent a great deal of time in the sauna – four hours a day for over two and a half weeks. I took vitamins and minerals and I prayed constantly. Through it all, I still believed the medical diagnosis that the doctors had given me was wrong, but in spite of everything I was doing to help myself, I remained very sick.

My biopsy result finally came back and the result was negative for bone cancer, which confused the doctors, since every test performed earlier had shown a tumour. The biopsy had, however, revealed dead cells along with normal bone cells. The test result was sent to the Mayo Clinic, where they determined that I had lymphatic cancer that had killed the cells in my femur. I knew this to be the truth and I believed mercury poisoning had caused it. How? I knew this because I had gone up and asked God (or the Creator) and had received the message that I had been poisoned by mercury.

I began to search for answers as to how to get the mercury out of my system. I continued with cleanses, always trusting in the information that I received from the Creator. By this time my leg had physically shrunk and I was told by the doctors that in the event that I did survive, I would need physical therapy to enable me to walk correctly again.

I believed to the core of my being that God could heal in an instant and in spite of everything that was happening, I continued to trust my intuition. Somehow I felt that I already knew how to heal myself. There was just something I was missing. I had used conventional medicine, cleanses, nutrition, oils, vitamins, affirmations and visualizations, and still I was sick. Every time I asked the Creator, I was told that I already knew the answer and that I just had to remember how to call upon God.

The answer to my prayers came while I was in the mountains. I held a gathering with some friends where we camped out and shared a pot luck dinner. Each person that came brought a dish for the gathering. My aunt from Oregon showed up unexpectedly, but had a bad stomachache. She lay down in a tent and I went inside to help her. She knew that I was a naturopath, but I had no herbs with me. The intense pain that she was in led me to believe that it might be her appendix. I began to do a body scan, as I had done with others hundreds of times before. I went out of the top of my head, through my crown chakra, as I would do when giving a reading, and when I was in my aunt's space I asked the Creator what was the matter with her and I was shown that it was giardia. I told it to go away and witnessed the Creator releasing the pain in her stomach. Within seconds, it had gone. She was able to get up and felt much better. This incident gave me food for thought and encouraged me to use it again.

The next day a man came into my practice with severe backache. Reflecting on what had happened with my aunt, I did the same procedure on him. Instantly, his back pain was gone.

That night, I pondered over the events of the past days. I decided it was time to do the same thing to myself.

The following day I hobbled into my office, excited at the prospect of carrying out the same procedure on my leg. I thought to myself, 'It can't be this easy!'

I stopped just before the door to my office and went out of my space from my crown chakra and prayed to the Creator. I then commanded a healing on myself, and it worked! My right leg, which had shrunk to three inches shorter than my left leg, returned instantly to its normal size. The pain was removed and my leg was healed.

I was so incredibly excited about my healing that throughout the day I compulsively tested the strength in my newly healed leg, curious to see if the pain would return.

Today my femur continues to be healthy, all test reports are normal and I am free of lymphatic cancer. In my gratitude I made a vow to the Creator to give this technique to all those who wanted to learn it. This was the foundation of the ThetaHealing that we know and love today.

Interestingly, I still have the X-rays of my leg. A few years ago, they were taken to a bone specialist for a second opinion and he pronounced that the owner of the leg must surely be dead!

The next person that I used the technique on was a little girl. A woman named Audrey Miller had a great-granddaughter with health difficulties and brought the child to me to be healed. She knew nothing about the instantaneous healing to my leg.

I asked her, 'Why did you bring her to me?'

Audrey looked at me with her soulful eyes and said, 'God told me to bring her to you.'

I remember how she walked up to me and placed the child in my arms. The child's own arms were tiny; she had gained no weight at all in the past two years. She had been born with her legs out of their sockets and she had a heart murmur. She also had what I can only term 'a bad attitude'.

I knew that I had been healed, so I told Audrey that it would take six days to heal the child, thinking that this would be plenty of time. I was excited about this new technique, but also very anxious. I remember crying to the Creator, 'Oh, dear Lord, please help me heal this child. Please, God, please, heal this child.' Then I went up to use the procedure I had been shown.

Each day for six days, Audrey's daughter drove for two hours to bring the child to me to be worked on for half an hour. I put her under coloured lights and used the new healing technique.

The little girl was using crutches to walk, the kind that attached to her arms. On the third day, she stood up and told me that she could walk and that she was going to walk to her grandmother without crutches. I said to her, 'Oh no, honey, you can't do that yet. You aren't strong enough.' But, stubbornly, she told me that she was going to do it. She stood up and walked about three or four feet to her grandmother. That was the first time she had ever walked on her own. I was totally amazed!

After that I watched her back straighten out and she expelled several tapeworms. Her heart murmur had now gone and she started, with physical therapy, to learn how to walk properly. Now that she had the strength, she could teach her body to walk without assistance. The most amazing part of this healing was that she gained two pounds in just three days, and in six days, she had gained four pounds.

Something was working! Excited, I began to use the technique on everyone. I treated all kinds of different diseases and infirmities and started working with people who were terminally ill. People from all walks of life found me by word of mouth. I found that the healings were extremely successful with clients that I already had and soon new clients were coming from all over the world. Many of them were healed instantly, while others took a few sessions, and others simply did not heal.

After using the procedure with varying degrees of success I came to a conclusion about why this technique was working so well. I came to believe that we were doing these healings from a 'Theta state' of mind. I had some knowledge of Theta because my by then former husband Blake was a hypnotist. He had many books about the subconscious mind and I had occasionally read these books. My theory was that we were going into the Theta state to bring about these healings. If my theory was correct, then I had a breakthrough in healing and an explanation of faith healing that could be scientifically measured.

2

THE FORMATION OF CLASSES

I knew that Theta was not a new theory of healing. Many hypnotists had actually worked with people in the Theta state. They had brought the client and also the health practitioner to a Theta state and achieved amazing results. I was also convinced that when you called upon God in this state, you could plug in, as if to an electrical socket, and actually heal a person instantly. I was already getting extremely good results, but I knew that it could be perfected if I had a better understanding of what I were doing, so I commenced investigating.

The human mind has five different brainwaves: Alpha, Beta, Gamma, Delta and Theta. These are constantly in motion; the brain is consistently producing waves in all of these frequencies. Everything that you do and everything you say is regulated by the frequency of your brainwaves.

A Theta state is a very deep state of relaxation, the state used in hypnosis. In Theta, the brainwaves are slowed to a frequency of four to seven cycles per second. Sages meditate for hours to reach this state, as in it they are able to access absolute calm. Theta brainwaves can be thought of as the subconscious; they govern the part of our mind that is layered between the conscious and the unconscious. They hold memories and sensations. They also govern our attitudes, beliefs and behaviour. They are always creative and inspirational and are characterized by very spiritual sensations. We believe this state allows us to act below the level of the conscious mind.

Theta is a very powerful state. It can be likened to the trance-like state that children attain when they are playing video games and are completely oblivious to what is going on around them. Another example of the use of Theta state is that of the Tibetan priests. In winter, these priests place wet towels over their shoulders. Within minutes the towels are completely dry. In ancient times the Kahunas of Hawaii accessed the Theta state to walk on hot lava.

·gan to teach this technique in the classes that I held locally.

my first class, a student stood up and told me that it was absolutely imposible to 'hold' a conscious Theta state. He said that he had been working with biofeedback for many years and unless a person was in a deep sleep hypnotic state, they just could not hold a Theta state. He claimed that the other brainwaves would interfere. He said that it was a great theory, but it was impossible. I was amused by his response and felt more determined than ever to prove my theory.

Validation for the Theta state came when a friend and student became interested in the work. He was a physicist who worked at the nuclear site outside town. He made us an electroencephalograph, and that's when things became interesting. In my classes, we hooked up people from all healing modalities to the machine. We found that people who were Reiki practitioners utilized the high Alpha brainwave. The Alpha brainwave is a wonderful healing wave. In fact, some Japanese scientists believe strongly in it because Alpha waves 'remove' pain and relax the body.

We confirmed that the technique we were using to do the healings was taking us to a Theta state. Every single person was going into Theta, even those just learning the technique. And we found that not only were the practitioners going into Theta, but the people they were working on were also going into Theta. We believed that the healings were taking place in a state of what I call 'God-consciousness'.

We continued to teach people as fast as we could. The classes were filled with wonderful people all eager to learn the technique. More and more people were learning and having a great time.

With continued practice, I found the healings became even more detailed and impressive. The results improved and my clientèle increased daily, but I still encountered a few people who would not heal.

One of those was a woman who had diabetes. Although her pain disappeared, her legs got better and so many other things improved for her, I could not keep her diabetes under control. Her blood sugar level still fluctuated dangerously. I knew that this type of diabetes was caused by a chromosome and I tried everything, even commanding the body to have its perfect blueprint. I was told that this did not work because the body thought it was perfect the way it was.

It was while working with this woman that I made a very interesting discovery. When I went 'up' and asked to see the chromosome that was causing her diabetes, in the rapture of Theta I was shown another chromosome that I was told was the chromosome of youth and vitality. Then I heard the voice of the Creator guiding me in a story of human DNA. I was told that this particular chromosome had been changed during the history of humankind's evolution. In a time and consciousness that is now lost to us, we were able to rejuvenate our body. We lost this ability over thousands of years, and because of this, this chromosome is now incomplete. However, in this time of enlightenment we are once again ready to receive regenerated youth.

I was told that the lost keys of youth and vitality in the DNA code were going to be vital to human survival in the years to come. This was, in part, because of the poisons and toxins that we would be subjected to in the modern industrial age. I was told that as a larger degree of the population became intuitive, they would become more sensitive to the physical world, but the completion of the youth and vitality chromosome would help them survive.

I was so excited about the new discovery that I forgot all about the chromosome for diabetes. I gave the woman with diabetes a hug, told her that I would work with her the next day and sent her home.

At the time, I was sharing my office with my friends Kevin and Chrissie. With glowing enthusiasm I told them all about what I had seen. I also told them that I had been given instruction on how to work on the chromosome and how to complete it. They were fascinated by the concepts and listened intently as I told them the process. I activated myself first and then Kevin and Chrissie. That evening I was given more information and guidance. In the coming days I was repeatedly shown how to change the youth and vitality chromosome until the Creator was sure that I had understood the information. This was the beginning of the DNA activation (see Chapter 26).

The Creator told me to begin with the DNA activation, activating the phantom DNA strands in a person's body. Understand that in this process we are not actually adding strands to anyone, we are only awakening what is already there. I was told that through this activation a person's intuition is improved, their ability to heal is improved, their body detoxifies and they are able to access the different planes of existence effortlessly. When I activated myself, I found that my 'laughter lines' began to fade away and my body started rejuvenating. I felt younger.

It was at this time that I hosted a radio talk show. I scheduled myself to speak about the Theta technique. When the radio staff asked me what it was called, I told them that I had always called it ThetaHealing. They advised me to choose another name because they felt that the name sounded like Scientology.

I told Kevin and Chrissie about this and we all sat down to brainstorm an alternate name. I remember us sitting on the floor of the office, laughing in our bare feet. I can still see Kevin with his long red hair and infectious laughter and Chrissie with her serious metaphysical demeanour. We remembered that the technique had been called many names. The first name I remembered was the Wilson technique, which was used for remote viewing in 1928. But we went even further back in time and Kevin and I agreed upon the name 'Orian' (with an 'a'). This was the name that we used: the Orian technique.

For the first few years I continued with this name, but ThetaHealing was more to my liking. Today we use the name 'ThetaHealing' for the brainwave Theta, originating from the Egyptian and Greek letter *theta*, meaning, among other things, 'soul'. The Orian technique was originally associated with the DNA activation, but ThetaHealing represents the complete healing modality, which stems from the thousands of readings, not to mention hundreds of classes and seminars, that I have done. Today both the names – 'Orian technique' and 'ThetaHealing' – are used, but ThetaHealing has become mainstream.

From the time of the talk show ThetaHealing began to take on a living essence of its own. Then I received a message from the Creator. In spite of all that was happening in my personal life, the Creator told me to take this information to the world and to share it with others. I told the Creator that I was the wrong person to do this. In fact, I spent several hours discussing it with the Creator. I had actually already given my word to take it to the world, but now the true ramifications of this responsibility were hitting home.

I remember reasoning with the Creator. I said, 'OK, if you want me to take this to the world, then send me a doctor, one who can tell me that this is the way a chromosome actually works, a doctor that will actually listen to me, a doctor who is open enough spiritually to listen to what I have to say. You also need to send me someone to write a book, because I am just too busy.'

I had many reasons for asking for all this. At that particular time in my life, my son's wife was pregnant and so was my daughter, and they were all living in my home. I was in the middle of a nasty divorce and I was taking care of all of these people by myself. I felt that my whole world was falling apart right before my eyes, and in the midst of all of this, I was being told by the Creator to take ThetaHealing to the world! I just couldn't understand how I could do any more than I was already doing.

So I was perplexed when the Creator said, 'You will write the book, Vianna.'

But I also knew that God never asks you to do anything without providing a way for you to do it.

Shortly thereafter, Audrey Miller came into my office quite unexpectedly and told me that I was going to the Universal Light Workers' Conference. I had seen the flyer for this and wanted to go, but I couldn't afford it.

But now this wonderful woman was willing to pay my fare and all of my expenses, including my food and everything else that I needed. She told me that I needed to meet a doctor that was speaking there. Apparently he was speaking about DNA. Audrey knew about the DNA activation that I was doing and thought that the two of us should meet. This was validation enough for me.

When it came near the time to go, however, I baulked, because I didn't want to leave my children at such a difficult time in their lives. The more I thought about it, the worse I felt. I made myself sick with anxiety. I was torn between staying and going. Needless to say, by the time I got to the conference, I was feeling pretty wrung out.

The first person that I met at the conference was the doctor I had asked God to show me. At the time he was doing extensive work with lasers and DNA. He seemed to be open-minded, so I tentatively began to tell him about what I was visualizing in the DNA activation. As we talked, he told me the names and functions of everything that I was seeing in the chromosomes – the shadow chromosomes, the telomeres – and he not only validated what I was seeing but said it was unlikely that I could have known some of this without having been instructed in some way. I told him that this was what God had shown me, and that inside the brain was the 'central cell' (so called by my friend Kevin) that was located in the pineal gland. This 'master cell' (as the doctor called it) is the creation point for sending messages to the rest of the body

I apparently piqued the doctor's curiosity. After our meeting he called on me to remote view clients as he visited them. He tested me with these people and asked me questions about what I could 'see' in their bodies. Then he not only confirmed what I had seen but his curiosity in my ability to 'see' what was going on in the body allowed me to know that I was viewing something real.

At the same conference I met Robert, who was a publisher. He had been involved with metaphysics before and as we talked he became interested in the DNA knowledge. We agreed that he should come to Idaho to transcribe the channelled material. I recorded the DNA activation technique for him and he and I agreed to co-author a small book. But when he took the recordings home to California, he wrote it and published it in pamphlet form, listing himself as the main author with my name in small print at the bottom. Much to my dismay, he changed the material so much and added so much filler that it had little to do with the original knowledge that I had given him. This book came out in 1997. This was a great disappointment to me and a betrayal of my trust; however, it encouraged me to rewrite the book and publish it myself.

By this time I felt that I could not trust anyone to compile a book on ThetaHealing, not even my closest friends. I decided to write the information down myself, in the form that it came to me from Creator, so that the vital points were not lost. God had once again worked in a strange way and I was guided by a divine plan. My first transcribed ThetaHealing book was called *Go Up and Seek God*.

True to my promise to the Creator, I began to teach classes throughout the United States in 1998. These were the first of the DNA 1 classes, where I taught the DNA activation and the early Orian Technique. In 1999, I created the first Teacher's Course to certify teachers in the Orian Technique. This was held at a place called Triple Creek in La Bell, Idaho. The course is now taught several times a year and I have been certifying teachers ever since. A *DNA 2 Teacher's Manual* was developed for it and is now updated constantly. The Creator was right; I would take the technique to the world.

I continued to see clients, and by the end of 1999 I had done over 20,000 readings and healings. As time went on I received more information and transcribed the book *Go Up and Work with God* in the year 2000. In this book, the belief work that came to me was put on paper for the first time. About this time, the DNA 1 Class (in what was then a two-day class) grew into what became known as DNA 2, a three-day class, in order to encompass the belief work. By the year 2000 I was teaching internationally.

One of the greatest things I have discovered while working on clients is that we hold the keys to our own health, our body and our vitality. The information I was given allows us to change our *beliefs*, and the systems that guide our decisions, in an instant. These are the beliefs and programmes we learned from childhood and from other aspects of our *being*. Some of them have been passed on from generation to generation.

In the following pages you will learn how to work on all four levels of all that you are: the *core belief level*, the *genetic level*, the *history level* and the *soul level*. It is through the removal and replacement of programmes on these four levels that the body is enabled to conquer physical illness and remove emotional blockage. This belief work will enable you to create the life that you want for yourself, for it is a truth that we create our own reality and that we are all connected to God. I am going to share with you the tools to change what you formerly believed, reverse the negative effect these beliefs have had on you and create the life you desire.

In the year 2000, a new class was shown to me called 'Psychic Anatomy'. I have since changed the name of this class to 'Intuitive Anatomy'. The first class was held at my old Channing Way, Idaho Falls, offices. It was designed to assist people to 'see' the inside of the body for healing, as an aid to the Theta technique. The body of knowledge of this class is held in the *Intuitive*

Anatomy Manual, published in 2003, and I now certify teachers for this class as well.

By the end of 2002, I had given almost 35,000 readings. The techniques that I learned in these sessions and classes are the foundations for this book.

In 2003, feeling work was added to the belief work. This was because I was told that certain people had never experienced particular feelings in their whole lives, nor did they understand how to create them. I was told that these feelings could be 'downloaded' into them from the Creator with their permission.

A considerable amount of knowledge was then collected and presented in the form of *The Advanced DNA 2 Class Manual*. In 2003, the first Advanced Class was held in Santa Rosa, California, and the first Advanced Teacher's Course was in 2004. This class was designed to get people ready for DNA 3 and to clarify the planes of existence, as will be explained further in this book. We will all be closer to DNA 3 when we have removed enough programmes and downloaded enough feelings to bring us to enlightenment.

The ThetaHealing 'tree' continues to grow as new information brings it into bloom. This book presents all the information compiled from the readings, healings and classes of ThetaHealing to date, from the instantaneous healing of my leg to the present day.

3

THE BASICS OF HEALINGS AND READINGS

I have been told by the Creator that long ago, in a time before written history, our intuitive abilities were much more advanced than they are now. Over aeons, many gifts have been lost. What we know today as ThetaHealing actually began thousands of years ago. I believe that these techniques are as old as time itself. They have been used for millennia as humanity awakens from time to time, only to fall asleep once more.

Now the long sleep is over and we are awake once again. I also believe that there is an inborn awareness in the human soul that will help us link this technique to ancient and future knowledge. In the past, genetics, energetic influences and collective consciousness issues kept us from developing to our full potential as Co-Creators with All That Is. We are now entering into a new transition of development. It is time to begin to accept our power as divine sparks of the Creator of All That Is.

THE FACETS OF THE JEWEL

Each aspect of ThetaHealing is like a facet of a jewel. Each facet works with all the others to make the jewel sparkle. Each person is like a jewel. Some are like diamonds in the rough that need to be polished. Others glitter even in the darkness. In this chapter we will discuss the aspects of ThetaHealing and how to harness them to make us shine.

The procedures for the basic healing and reading techniques of ThetaHealing are really quite easy to follow. However, for the person that has not opened themselves to their true intuitive potential, the *modus operandi* of these techniques, visualization, is something that may not come naturally. So some people must practise this technique first. What we have found, however, is that everyone can learn it. If you follow the instructions at your own pace you will become skilled at it.

Healings and readings are based upon the power of controlled and focused *thought*. In order to control and focus thought we must learn all that we can of our inherent potential. In order to understand the process, you must first recognize your own intuitive abilities.

Perhaps some of you will have heard of these terms, but others will have not. These are the first 'branches' of the ThetaHealing 'tree' we use to 'go up and seek God':

1. The power of words and thoughts.
2. The brainwaves.
3. The psychic senses and chakras.
4. Free agency, co-creation.
5. The power of observation and being the witness.
6. The command.
7. The Creator of All That Is.

Once you understand these topics you will be guided through the first technique.

Note: Throughout the text you will see the symbol for Theta, Θ, used to mark an important notation.

THE POWER OF WORDS AND THOUGHTS

In ThetaHealing, we work with the Creator of All That Is. We explore the subconscious and the conscious mind. These elements of our mind are each incredibly powerful in their own way.

One of the things that you must remember when you are working with the subconscious mind is that you have to use words the subconscious understands. One of the concepts that the subconscious mind does *not* understand is the word 'try'. You cannot *try* to do anything. You cannot *try* to pick up a pencil; it just can't be done. You either do it or you don't do it. In fact, if you say to your friend, 'I'll try to be there,' you might as well say that you are *not* going to be there. I could tell my children, 'Tidy your rooms.' If they tell me, 'I will *try* to!', I know that it will never happen. Since the subconscious does not understand the word 'try', it just assumes that whatever it is doesn't have to be done. So, you are not going to *try* these techniques; you are going to *experience* them. Absolutely eliminate the word 'try'. Instead, say, 'I'm going to use this technique. I'm going to *do* it.' Approach this with a 'do' attitude.

As a ThetaHealing practitioner, you will develop the ability to create manifestations with the power of the spoken word and the formed thought.

15

The belief that the spoken utterance and thought forms have power to create physical changes is as old as the sentience of humans. The things that we say and especially our thought forms are magnified by the use of ThetaHealing. This is because when we are in Theta, we connect not only to our own divinity but also directly to the Divine, the Creator of All That Is. It is therefore important for you to be constantly aware of any random thoughts or utterances. Some examples of negative thought forms and spoken words are:

- 'I need to lose weight.' (If you lose it you will always be looking for it.)
- 'I can't afford it.' (You will never afford anything, or have abundance, since you can't afford it.)
- 'Money is the root of all evil.' (If money is evil then you will always shun money and opportunities for money.)

Words, either spoken out loud or voiced in thought form, have an incredible effect upon our daily life. If a statement is made enough times, it becomes a reality. If thoughts are in a deep enough Theta-wave, instant manifestations are possible. This is especially true if we are in the pure and meditative Theta state of mind that connects us to the Creator of All That Is. Interestingly, science is now coming out of the imperialism of its own dark ages and is exploring the possibilities of the power of *thought*.

Think about all the thought forms and words that are in your paradigm. What do they mean to you on all levels of your being? Perhaps they are blocking you from progressing without your knowing it. As you develop your intuitive abilities with ThetaHealing, words, thought forms and belief systems will all have the power to create changes in your daily life for good or ill.

CELLULAR COMMUNICATION

A good example of the power of thought has been revealed in research done with plants. Some time ago a brilliant researcher named Cleve Backster decided to test the response capability of a dracaena plant by hooking it up to the galvanic skin response section of a polygraph. He was amazed when he got a human-like reading from the plant. Later in the observation period he found that the chart showed the dracaena reacting wildly to his intention to threaten its well-being by burning it, at the very moment that the thought occurred to him.

After also discovering response capability in yogurt bacteria, algae, yeast and food, Backster separated human white cells (leukocytes) from saliva and placed millions of them in a test tube wired to an EEG via electrodes. The donor was at a distance of 20 or more miles, but the cells reacted to the donor's stress or arousal at exactly the same time.

If we can send a microwave through the air that permits us to communicate via mobile phones, it stands to reason that our brain can act in a similar way. This is why we must be careful of all the thought forms in our mind. Our experience of life will be as positive or negative as our thoughts, because thoughts have real substance.

When we are in a deep Theta state, our thoughts and words become much more powerful. When someone speaks directly to you, with something such as, 'Are you feeling OK? You don't look well!' it is up to you, with *free agency*, whether or not you accept or decline this suggestive thought. If you accept it, you could become ill – or tired, sad, happy, full of energy, etc., depending upon the suggestive statement.

Similarly, be very careful of the thought forms that are directed toward you and your acceptance of them. As your intuition deepens, you will become aware of them.

Words and thought forms become magnified when in Theta state. By holding a conscious Theta state you can create anything and change reality instantly.

BRAINWAVES

To understand the Theta state, you must first understand brainwaves.

There are five different frequencies of brainwave: Beta, Alpha, Theta, Delta and Gamma. These are constantly in motion since the brain is consistently producing waves in all frequencies. Everything that you do and say is regulated by the frequency of your brainwaves and one frequency will dominate in any given situation.

BETA

Whenever you are thinking, talking and communicating, your mind is in Beta. It will be in Beta at this moment. Beta waves have a frequency of 14–28 cycles per second. Beta is the state in which you are active and alert.

ALPHA

Alpha is the bridge between Beta and Theta. In an Alpha state, your brainwaves are moving at a frequency between 7 and 14 cycles per second.

The Alpha frequency is likened to a very relaxed, meditative state of mind. Alpha waves govern daydreaming and fantasizing, and denote relaxed, detached awareness.

People who don't function well at this frequency will experience memory difficulties. For example, if you are aware that a particular dream or meditation was quite powerful, but can't recall the details, sufficient Alpha frequencies were not generated. You didn't have the bridge between the subconscious and the conscious mind.

To more fully understand an Alpha state, close your eyes and imagine a sunset. See in your mind's eye the sun setting against the ocean and seagulls flying low near the shore. This is the beginning of inducing an Alpha state.

When we tested Reiki energy healers on an electroencephalograph, we found that they that they were using the Alpha brainwave. In Reiki, the practitioner brings the 'Source' into their body. The energy is then manipulated through the hands to heal a person. The electroencephalograph showed that when Source-energy came into the healer's body and into the hands to heal, their brain was in an Alpha state. Alpha has been known to take away pain and is useful in healing.

THETA

A Theta state is a very deep state of relaxation. This is the state used in hypnosis and dreaming. In it, the brainwaves are slowed to a frequency of four to seven cycles per second. In fact, sages meditate for hours and hours to reach this state, as in it they are able to access absolute calmness.

Theta brainwaves can be thought of as the subconscious; they govern the part of our mind that is layered between the conscious and the unconscious. They hold memories and sensations. They also govern our attitudes, beliefs and behaviour. They are always creative, inspirational and characterized by very *spiritual* sensations.

It is believed the Theta state allows us to act below the level of the conscious mind. It is the first stage of the dream state. It is the state we are in when we stand on the top of a mountain completely absorbed in our surroundings. At that moment of realization we experience the absolute 'knowing' that God is real; we just know that God *is*. When we access a Theta state and call upon the Creator, we connect to the Creator of All That Is to heal a person instantly.

In ThetaHealing, when you imagine yourself going up above your head through your crown chakra, your brain will still be in an Alpha state on the electroencephalograph. But it has been shown that when consciousness is sent through the crown with the focused thought that it will *go up and seek God*, the brain automatically shifts to a pure *Theta state* on the electroencephalograph. What did the ancients mean when they said, 'Go up and ask of God?' When you imagine lifting your consciousness above your head through your crown chakra and you go up and ask of God, your brainwaves shift instantly to Theta.

When I was asked what I was doing in my readings, this is what I realized. I was sitting across from the person, holding their hands and imagining myself going above my space, praying that God would grant me the reading that this person needed, and it was given to me. I was holding a Theta state.

DELTA

A Delta state of mind happens when you are in a deep sleep. In a Delta state, the brainwaves are slowed to a frequency of zero to four cycles per second. It is also this state that is utilized when the phone rings and we intuitively 'know' who is calling.

GAMMA

The Gamma brainwave is the state we are in when we learn and process information. Gamma waves stimulate the release of Beta endorphins. They appear to be involved in higher mental activity, including perception and consciousness. In this state, your brainwaves cycle between 40 and 5,000 cycles a second.

I believe that when you are in a Theta-Gamma state, you are in the condition most conducive to instant healing. In the miracle of instant healing the brain can go from 4 cycles a second to 5,000 cycles a second.

In times of emergency, the brain has been observed to switch back and forth between Gamma and Theta with no other wave present. This seems to be a natural response.

Gamma waves disappear when a person is under anaesthesia. They may be involved in binding a variety of sensory inputs into the single unitary object we perceive. Recordings of neurons in the visual cortex show that synchronization in the Gamma band links parts of the cortex excited by the same object and not those excited by different objects, implicating Gamma rhythms in binding. For instance, the colour, shape, movement and location of an object are processed in different ways in the visual cortex, and these features of an object need to be reunited into a single entity. This is known as the binding problem (which may be the reason why people accumulate free-floating memories in an unconscious state), and Gamma rhythms are thought to provide a solution. In fact, this process is so efficient that we are hardly aware that it goes on at all.

BRAINWAVES AND HEALING

Scientists have discovered that certain brain frequencies (particularly in the Alpha, Theta and Theta-Gamma states) have been found to do the following:

- alleviate stress and promote a long-lasting and substantial reduction in anxiety
- facilitate deep physical relaxation and mental clarity
- increase verbal ability and verbal performance IQ
- synchronize both hemispheres of the brain
- invoke vivid spontaneous mental imagery and imaginative creative thinking
- reduce pain, promote euphoria and stimulate endorphin release

Findings from a recent study reported in the *American Journal of Psychiatry* suggest that increased Theta-wave activity in prefrontal brain regions is related to medication-free recovery from symptoms of major depression. Leuchter and colleagues (2002) found that increases in quantitative electroencephalography (QEEG) cordance measures of Theta-wave activity (four to eight Hz) were positively associated with clinical response to a 'sugar pill'.[1]

In this study, no statistically significant differences were found between response rates to antidepressant medication and a placebo. However those patients who responded to medication did exhibit decreased prefrontal Theta cordance (PTC), whereas placebo responders showed increased PTC. Patients who did not respond to either treatment did not show any significant changes in PTC. Thus, increases in PTC appear to be uniquely associated with symptom improvement in patients receiving a placebo – a 'no drug' condition.

The effectiveness of placebo treatment is thought to depend, in part, on the patient's expectation that they will get better. In double-blind clinical trials such as this one, neither patients nor their doctors know who is receiving the medication and who the placebo until the end of the study.

---

1. Leuchter, A. F., Cook, I. A., Witt, E. A., Morgan, M., and Abrams, M., 'Changes in brain function of depressed subjects during treatment with placebo', *American Journal of Psychiatry* 159 (2002), 122–9 (submitted by Aimee M. Hunter, PhD, NIMH Research Fellow)

Patients taking placebos often believe that they are taking active medication and often believe that the treatment will work. So, increase in frontal lobe Theta activity, seen in the placebo response, may reflect a physiological mechanism related to natural (medication-free) healing from depression.

THE PSYCHIC SENSES

The electrical energy of the brainwaves has a direct connection with what are traditionally called the 'psychic senses'. In order for the mind to hold the deep meditative state of Theta, all of the psychic senses and the chakras (energy centres) must be in union, or in what the ancients called *kundalini*.

There are different intuitive or psychic senses that are inherently active in many people and yet in others are asleep, waiting to awaken. Many people have these intuitive senses buried under layers of *belief systems*. In the Theta state they are awakened and brought together to coalesce in one consciousness that is sent to seek God.

These are the different senses:

EMPATHY

The empathic sense is located in the solar plexus, roughly between the ribs and the stomach.

This is the quality of experiencing another person's feelings by projecting our electromagnetic field on an instinctual level or connecting with what they are feeling. We understand this to mean that we each have our own sense of 'feeling' of how another person experiences emotional thought forms on a spiritual, mental, physical or metaphysical level.

An example of the empathic ability would be when someone has a stomachache and you feel the same pain, to a lesser extent, in your own stomach. You simply 'know' that the person has difficulties there. The empathic sense also enables you to know instantly how people feel about you when you enter a room, to sense whether you are liked or disliked.

CLAIRVOYANCE

When engaging our clairvoyant senses we use the energy of the third eye, in the centre of the brow, in correspondence with the other centres of the body.

Clairvoyance is the ability to see objects or events that are not perceived by the everyday senses. It is 'second sight', using the visualization of the mind's eye to see auric energy and visions of events. Some clairvoyants also have the ability to read the thoughts of other people using telepathy.

Being clairvoyant enables you to see into the body. When you become clairvoyantly developed, you will get very accurate body readings. The third eye is accurate when you are reading a person's body because it deals with the here and now, but it is not as accurate for predicting the future, because when you use it you invariably tell a person what they want to hear rather than what they should hear. That is because with this ability we see the future through the person's greatest fears and desires, and this may not necessarily be the greatest *truth* for that person. For example, someone may be afraid that they have cancer everywhere in their body. When an intuitive uses only the third eye, they may 'read' that fear, instead of the truth. For the greatest truth, you must first connect with the Creator of All That Is.

CLAIRAUDIENCE

The clairaudient sense is our auditory system. It is located above our ears.

This is the ability to hear sounds or speech not perceived by the everyday sense of hearing. It is the last of the psychic senses to develop. This is the one that enables us to hear our guardian angels as well as other auditory messages.

An example of this would be hearing your guardian angels speaking to you in a tone of warning, saying, '*Stop!* Don't cross the street!' These voices are not always heard with our ears, but can be heard as a thought form or even as a vibration all around us.

PROPHECY

This is the ability to reveal or predict with certainty using divine inspiration. By creating a connection with the Divine, we become prophetic.

In the power of the prophetic, we learn to combine all the psychic senses to access pure Theta brainwaves. To engage our prophetic senses, we send our consciousness to our crown chakra and go up through all the planes to connect to the Creator of All That Is and make the command. We are then able to become all that we can be as an intuitive person. The crown chakra is called the *prophetic chakra* because it is where the abilities of the Divine begin to open.

The psychic senses relate directly to the timeless concept of the chakras, the energy potentials wherein the psychic senses reside.

THE CHAKRAS

Volumes can be, and have been, written about the chakras. They are energy centres that lie along the axis of the spine as consciousness potentials. Interestingly, each of them correlates to major nerve ganglia branching forth from the spinal column. The psychic senses reside within these whirling vortexes of energy.

The concept of the chakras, or 'energy centres' in the body, pervades, in some form, many cultures around the world. However, no culture developed the idea more than the Hindu, from Tantric philosophy and Yoga.

The chakras are not to be understood as real in the physical sense but as situated in the auric body. They are repositories of intuitive energies. In the Hindu religion they are usually represented as blossoming lotuses. In ThetaHealing there are exercises to open and use these intuitive energy centres.

KUNDALINI

The spiritual person is on a quest for *kundalini* energy. When it comes to pass, the intuitive is awakened with new enlightenment.

The *Shakti*, or female energy, resides at the base of the spine. She begins to flow up through the body, opening each chakra as she ascends, until she merges with the *Shiva*, or male essence, in the *sahasrara* chakra. The Shiva and the Shakti aspects in a person's spiritual essence then merge, creating balance.

As *kundalini* energy reaches each chakra, each 'lotus' opens and lifts its flower. As soon as the energy moves to a higher chakra, the lotus closes its petals and hangs down, symbolizing the activation of the energies of the chakra and their integration into the *kundalini*.

In the Theta technique, a person draws the *kundalini* energy from the centre of the Earth and ignites each chakra as the energy flows up the body to the crown chakra. As the consciousness goes out of the crown chakra, the person is balanced with the *kundalini* energy and the consciousness can then go up to the Creator as a *balanced* spiritual essence. (*This is further explained in Chapter 6.*)

The Theta state of mind is obtained when you send out your consciousness to connect to the Creator through the crown chakra. Although all the chakras are used in readings, it is the crown chakra that is the most prevalent in ThetaHealing, as this is the 'gateway' to the Creator's truth.

When we consider truth, the concept of *free agency* opens our potential not only to use our inherent abilities but also to co-create with the Creator of All That Is.

FREE AGENCY, CO-CREATION

It is important to consider the concept of freedom as it relates to meditation and prayer for the individual. Free will and free agency are beliefs that we have the power to make our own choices. The spiritual connotations of free agency give us the self-authority to connect to what we perceive to be God or the Creator. In ThetaHealing, we have free agency to connect the inner and outer aspects of the Divine within ourselves to that which is outside ourselves.

As we move through this existence we are given opportunities to create some of our own pathways to find our way. We are given the tools of *morals* and *respect* for others, but the Creator loves us enough to also give us the opportunity to experience the joy of life without interference or judgement. Our existence here can be perceived as a beautiful learning experience of physical, mental and spiritual exploration.

It is through the gift of *co-creation* or *synergy with God* that it is possible to bring the Creator into our reality to heal others and ourselves. We unite with the Creator and become the *witness*.

THE POWER OF OBSERVATION AND BEING THE WITNESS

In a deep Theta wave, we open doorways to healings, readings and manifestations. It is therefore necessary for us to *witness* the healing energy of the Creator until the full process has finished. Nothing happens in nature without it being 'seen' or 'witnessed'. Our mind does not accept something as real until it has been formed as a burning vision. When it becomes a vision, it is accepted as real to us as well as to the Creator. This is why developing visualization skills is so important.

Everyone visualizes. However, some people think that this means that they see the visualization behind their eyelids. This is incorrect. The place where the visualization is seen is the place where we envision our memories. Some people call this 'feeling'. People often get mixed up with what is 'feeling' and what is seeing. If you *feel* a colour is green, then you are *visualizing* it. Similarly, a person might say, 'I feel you have a spot on your liver.' This is also a form of visualization and the person would do well to develop this process.

Visualization is in fact an action that we carry out every minute of every day. Ninety per cent of the brain's sensory input is visual and at least half of the stored memory is visual as well. So we visualize constantly, whether we are aware of it or not.

We use the imagery in our mind's eye to plan and conduct our life. When you set out to go to a destination, for example, whether it is familiar or not, your mind pictures the place and the route to get there. Before going to a place you have not been before, you plan your way beforehand. How? You use your imagination. You use your ability to visualize. You visualize the road, the streets you have to pass through, and even the traffic lights. If someone were to ask you how to get to a destination, you would describe the way, while at the same time you would see the route in your imagination.

Whenever you decide to mow the lawn, cook dinner, buy a new dress, clean your home, tell a joke or describe a book or film, imagination and visualization are at work. The eye of the mind is constantly in motion.

Let's take daydreams, for example. Here we imagine scenarios and actions in the movie of the mind. And at the moment that we daydream, the daydream becomes real to us. If we repeat the same daydream over a period of time it becomes a habit. We may even start to believe it and accept it as a reality, especially when strong emotions are involved.

Expecting the vision to become reality is more than just an act of visualization, it is an act of *creation*. Deciding upon something that we really want to happen and visualizing it with concentration, faith and desire sets great powers in motion. The creation of reality through visualization is a natural process that all of us unconsciously employ. Thoughts that pass through our mind create our life. It is only the *perception* of imagination and reality that cause some people confusion.

Seeing pictures in your mind's eye is the mental tool that is used in ThetaHealing. Close your eyes now and 'see' a view of nature, a sunset for example. It is in this place that we will view the inside of the body to see any difficulties.

The development of visualization is easy once you familiarize yourself with it. And as you practise the technique, *all* the intuitive skills will develop. Your feeling, auditory and visualization skills will develop in synchronicity with one another. This will make you an awesome instrument of the Creator.

The brain is like a muscle. The more we develop it, the better it becomes at doing something. The more we connect to the Creator, the better we will become at seeing inside the body, performing healing and being the witness. Once we connect with the Creator imagination becomes real.

Remember that there is no such thing as not being able to visualize. If you are 'remote viewing' in someone's body and are having a difficult time visualizing, you may be imagining yourself too close to or too far away from the affected area to see it. Move your mind like the focus on a camera closer or farther away to see the affected area clearly. Becoming more familiar with anatomy can reduce confusion as to what you are seeing while in the body, giving a focal point of reference for the vision so you know where you are. Being familiar with anatomy also prevents your mind from using the excuse that it cannot understand the inner realm of the human body.

> *When we have discussed belief work in later chapters, test yourself for negative programmes on the belief levels pertaining to visualization and release any negative programmes that you might have.*

> Θ *As a practitioner of ThetaHealing, it is important to learn visualization skills to bring healing into reality. You witness the healing coming to pass.*

IMAGINATION

While visualizing in a Theta state, it is your imagination that you are using. Most people do not know the dictionary definition of imagination:

1. *The ability to visualize; The ability to form images and ideas in the mind, especially of things never seen or never experienced directly.*
2. *Creative part of the mind; The part of the mind where ideas, thoughts, and images are formed.*
3. *Resourcefulness; The ability to think of ways of dealing with difficulties or problems.*
4. *Creative act; An act of creating a semblance of reality, especially in literature.*

I realize that at first visualizing will seem as though it's all 'in your imagination', but in truth, imagination is using your subconscious mind and the Theta wave. The subconscious mind is in charge of memory and feelings; the conscious mind is in charge of decisions.

THE COMMAND

In ThetaHealing, when we go up out of our space and connect to the Creator to start the co-creation process, we use the word 'command' in the prayer that is spoken to the Creator. For example:

'It is commanded that unconditional love is sent through every cell of this person's body. Thank you! It is done. It is done. It is done.'

It is important that you understand the use and meaning of the word 'command', or a command statement such as 'Creator, show me.' The definitions of 'command' are as follows:

To overlook.

To have at one's disposal, e.g. command of a language.

To deserve and receive due observance.

A signal to activate.

Sub-words in the word 'command':

Co: In Latin the meaning is an intensive 'with', as in 'co-operate'.

Com: To invite to unite or join with, as in 'come'.

Man: Creator. Found in other words such as:

Manifesto: Public declaration of intent or principles.

Manifold: Multiply, of many kinds, a whole made up of diverse elements.

Mandala: A design symbolizing the universe.

Mandible: The lower part of jaw, which is necessary in speaking; we create with words.

Mandare: (Latin) to order.

As you can see, the word 'command' is all about empowering you with an understanding of the Creator.

It is interesting to compare it to the word 'demand': *de* in the Latin form means 'oppose, reverse, remove, reduce'.

When you use the word 'command' in the statement to God, Creator, Source, or however you feel comfortable naming Divinity, several things happen that transcend a simple prayer. In making the command, there is no question in your mind that the statement will be done, since this process removes all doubts and disbeliefs as to your own worthiness, power or otherwise. If 'I command' sounds too selfish to you, then say, 'It is commanded.'

Once you are used to making the command in a healing, the use of a spontaneous thought form of 'commanding energy' will be sufficient and the process will be as swift as thought and needs only to be witnessed.

In making the command, you permit the Creator of All That Is into the quotient, without the interference of the human factor. When the command has been made and accepted, you are free to play the role of the witness in the healing process and the Creator is free to perform the healing.

When you first make the command it is important that it is done silently, at least at first. The reason for this is that for most people it is difficult to hold a Theta state while speaking aloud. As you practise, however, you will be able to hold a Theta state when speaking aloud.

Θ *Remember, there is more than one way to envision or address the Creator of All That Is. Use the word that makes you feel the most comfortable. The name with which you make the command must pertain to your belief system, not to another person's perceptions of what God is or is not. Buddha, Shiva, Goddess, Jesus, Yahweh and Allah are all currents leading in a flow towards the Seventh Plane of Existence and the Creative Energy of All That Is.*

4

THE ROAD MAP TO ALL THAT IS

In retrospect, I can see that when I first began to seriously conduct readings and healings, a doorway was somehow opened for me. In a way, I was a little like Alice in Wonderland when she tumbled down the rabbit hole. I began to have metaphysical experiences that increased in intensity. As I have explained, I have always been intuitive and have what some call 'the sight'. But there was little to prepare me for what was to come.

I suspect that my intuitive senses began to open fully as information began to flood into my mind from what I came to know as the planes of existence. In these early experiences I met the Law of Truth, who taught me the concept of the seven planes of existence. (*The seven planes of existence will be fully explained in Chapter 16.*) The seven planes provided me with a conceptual medium for understanding how and why the world works on the physical and spiritual levels and how this relates to us as humans. This gave me a better understanding of the concept of the Creator of All That Is. I learned that through the Creator of All That Is, it is possible to create physical healing, to progress spiritually and to find enlightenment. The more that I made a direct connection to the Creator of All That Is from the Seventh Plane, the clearer my perspective became of the other planes of creation that make up the whole.

Conveying a process that occurs within the realm of the metaphysical can be a challenge. Our verbal language has no words for much of the pure transpirations of spiritual thought forms and spiritual information. It is even more challenging to convey these experiences via the written word. Since the invention of writing, holy people, prophets and seers have attempted to put spiritual concepts into word and onto paper, but the expression of concepts that are a *pure vibration* has a tendency to fall short of the original purity of the Divine.

When I first began to teach others what I was doing with Theta, I came to realize that the process was so spontaneous that the spoken and written word could not easily do it justice. But somehow I had to bring a spiritual concept into words, since words were all that I had!

The first attempt to teach people what I was doing in readings was to 'release people from their paradigm'. I used a meditational process to send their consciousness 3, 6 or 67 feet above themselves to connect to God. In my early books, *Go Up and Seek God* and *Go Up and Work with God*, I used this 3, 6 or 67 feet as the early road map to the highest energy. This process of meditation was designed to release the consciousness from the magnetic pull of the Earth and the egoism of the person.

At the time, I thought that this was as good a way as any I had been given to connect others to the Creator of All That Is. But, as I taught, I found that people had many limiting belief systems. So the process was successful with some people but not with all of them. Some people would become confused, others needed to be counselled as I took them through the process and still others went to places that were dictated by their misleading beliefs.

Some of my students began to ask me what I was doing differently when I went up to connect to the Creator. It seems that they instinctively knew that I was going somewhere that they were not. I had been doing the process for so long that it had become instantaneous for me. After serious consideration I sat down in meditation to discover if I was going somewhere different from the 3, 6 or 67 feet out of my space that I had been teaching. I took the time to reflect upon just what I was doing and how I could put it into words for others to benefit from. This is the process that came to me and how I learned to part the veil.

GO UP TO THE CREATOR OF ALL THAT IS OF THE SEVENTH PLANE!

The following process was given to me by the Creator to train All That You Are to connect to and understand All That Is. Once this is learned, you will consistently go to the Seventh Plane and you will not need to go through the whole process, you will simply be there.

Imagine energy coming up through the bottom of your feet from the centre of the Earth and going up out of the top of your head as a beautiful ball of light. You are in this ball of light. Take time to notice what colour it is.

Now imagine going up above the universe.

Now imagine going into the light above the universe. It is a big be
light.

Imagine going up through that light, and you'll see another bright light, and another, and another. In fact there are many bright lights. Keep going. Between the lights there is a little bit of dark light, but this is just a layer before the next light, so keep going.

Finally there is a great big bright light. Go through it. When you go through it, you're going to see an energy, a jelly-like substance that has all the colours of the rainbow in it. When you go into it you see that it changes colour. This is the Laws. You will see all kinds of shapes and colours.

In the distance, there is a white iridescent light; it is a white-blue colour, like a pearl. Head for that light. Avoid the deep blue light, because this is the Law of Magnetism.

As you get closer, you may see a mist of a pink colour. Keep going until you see it. This is the Law of Compassion, and it'll push you into the special place.

You will see that the pearlescent light is the shape of a rectangle, like a window. This window is really the opening to the Seventh Plane. Now go through it. Go deep within it. See a deep, whitish glow go through your body. Feel it. It feels light, but it has essence. You can feel it going through you; it's as if you can no longer feel the separation between your own body and the energy. You become All That Is. Don't worry. Your body will not disappear. It will become perfect and healthy. Remember there is just energy here, not people or things. So if you see people, go higher.

It is from this place that the Creator of All That Is can perform instant healing and that you can create in all aspects of your life.

An alternative method is as follows:

Seat yourself in a comfortable chair or sofa and take a deep breath in. Imagine that you and the chair have become as one on a molecular level. Your molecules and that of the chair are transferring back and forth between one another. You are not stretching, but rather connecting to the molecules, becoming as one.

Now imagine that on a molecular level you are a part of everything in the room. Expand outward and become as one with the outside world.

Imagine that you are a part of the area, then the country that you are in.

Imagine that you are a part of the entire Earth, connecting to earth, land and sea, every creature, every nation on this planet, until you and the Earth are one and the same.

Imagine that you and the universe are one and the same.

Imagine that you are a part of all the bright white lights.

Imagine that you are a part of the jelly-like substance.

Finally imagine that you are a part of an iridescent white light that is the Seventh Plane of Existence. Become as one with this iridescent white light.

Take a deep breath in and open your eyes. Welcome to the Seventh Plane of Existence. For behold, you are not separate, you are a part of God – All That Is.

> Θ *People naturally resist moving out of their comfort zone. It may take some time to train your brain to go to the Seventh Plane of Existence. If you find that you have an issue with this process, ask the Creator to take you to the Seventh Plane of Existence to the Creative Energy of All That Is. It is your birthright to use this energy.*
>
> *You may also like to try meditating to reach the Seventh Plane (see page 34).*

The process of going up to the Seventh Plane will unlock doors in your mind to connect you with All That Is. It seems to connect the neurons in your brain back to the point of *creation*. In fact, after you have truly gone to the Seventh Plane and you open your eyes you will realize that you are connected to *everything* and that the veil has been lifted.

When the true connection to the Creator is made, you may feel a tingling on the top of the head. You will know when you connect to the Creator. The connection just is.

> Θ *Remember, it is not your spirit that is going up to the Seventh Plane, only a consciousness that is created by the process.*

Repeatedly perform this process step by step before you use a shortcut to command that you be taken to the Seventh Plane.

When you go to the Seventh Plane using this process, the perception is that you are going outside yourself, out into the universe to the far reaches of the cosmos and through a portal into creation. In a way this is true, but not the way that you might think. Inside every person there is a tiny universe that is identical to the vastness of All That Is.

So, what do we find inside ourselves? We find that inside each of us there is the Creative Force, Source and God. *Infinity* is inside us as well as outside. So where are you going when you go up and seek God? Where are you going when you go through the jelly-like substance? You are entering the nucleus of an atom. Each time that you connect to the Creator, you go on a journey in the inner vastness. This journey connects you to your own atoms and also brings you to the awareness of the *outside* universe of infinite energy and to the realization that God is in every atom.

So you go on a journey inside yourself to find the Creator-self that is inside you and outward to the cosmic consciousness.

COSMIC CONSCIOUSNESS

Cosmic consciousness is very different from our earthly awareness. There are many perceptions that are specific aspects of this world. Many of these are purely of a human design, while others have been created following divine inspiration. It can be difficult to perceive which concepts are of this Earth, which are illusions, which are those we have created and which are divine. For instance, human collective consciousness has not yet developed sufficiently to be purely divine. It has a competitive streak running through it that is not only part of our perception but is in our very DNA. Reincarnation is another example of the many concepts that exist on planet Earth as a consciousness but not necessarily a purely *divine* perception.

This is why it is so important that our perceptions are as pure as possible and why we leave this earthly illusion to be with the Creator to create healing. By taking the road map out past the stars into creation we break through the earthly bounds that hold us to become a cosmic power that is not bound by the Laws of Earth.

These are some of the aspects and perceptions that are released when we use the road map to the Seventh Plane of Existence:

- the human ego
- death
- physical and mental emotions (for example, fear, doubt and disbelief)
- group consciousness

- dualism
- instinctual desires
- passions
- being human in a physical world
- the illusion of the physical
- having to suffer (suffering is a choice)
- having to sacrifice (sacrifice is a choice)
- being separate
- the need for 'brain candy'

DAILY THETAHEALING MEDITATION

Utilize this meditation daily to practise being connected to All That Is. The longer you hold this energy, the easier it is to create good things in your life.

Imagine energy coming up from the centre of the Earth into the bottom of your feet, going up to the top of your head and going above your space in a beautiful ball of light. Passing all the planes of existence, you go directly to the Seventh Plane, and poof, you're there.

When you get to the Seventh Plane, the ball of light that surrounds you disappears and the energy of All That Is envelopes each and every molecule and atom that makes you who you are until finally you dissolve into the love of the Creator of All That Is. There is no fear. You just gently feel this energy moving through everything. You realize that you're a part of everything and everyone.

It's easy to manifest in this energy because you realize that you're a part of everybody and everything that is. You can feel the energy all around you, and as you realize this, your body comes into perfect balance.

Now is the time to think about what it is that you want in your life. Imagine that it is sitting in your life already and that you are a part of it. Take a deep breath in and open your eyes, feeling totally connected to All That Is. It is from this place that you're connected to All That Is, feeling that you can change the outcomes and energy in your life.

This is the ascension to All That Is. Throughout the book this will be the navigation process to the Creator of All That Is.

5

THE READING

Now that you have the background information regarding this technique, we will put all the pieces together for the reading. The most important part for you to understand is that *you* have the ability to do everything I teach you. With practice, *everyone* has this ability; *anyone* can do it. Please keep in mind that the concepts that are discussed in this book are *real*. They work, and they work because you are accessing a brainwave that places you in a meditative state that allows you to make contact with the Creator of All That Is.

Perhaps I should say that you are simply being *reminded* of this knowledge, because on some level you are already familiar with it. Remember, we are all *divine* in nature and it is our divine perception of God that is our Source of Divinity.

The most important thing that you must have when you are doing readings, or doing any of these techniques, is a belief in God. It doesn't matter what belief system you embrace; what is important is that your beliefs work *for* you, not *against* you. We must stay with the *truth*: that we are all connected to the whole. It is this whole, this completeness, this God that we call upon in doing this work.

While you are in a person's body, silently and gently looking around, you are in what is called a prophetic or healing state. When you are in this state you have the ability to see truth. As you speak and tell the person what you see, your brainwaves begin to go back up to Beta. Any time you speak aloud, your brainwaves will go back up to Beta, but once you become silent again you will return to Theta. This process teaches the mind to automatically shift from Beta to Alpha to Theta, back to Alpha then back to Beta on command.

The very act of commanding a reading will usually put the receiver into a Theta state along with the practitioner. As the client is receiving the healing, they need to remain quiet and calm. So, tell the person to relax and close their eyes. As already mentioned, it is very difficult for some people to hold a Theta brainwave while speaking out loud, so say the command process mentally to yourself. Each time you speak to the client and then become silent again, you will automatically go back and forth from Beta to Theta. Renewing the silence will place you firmly back into the Theta wave each time you answer any questions or continue any processes.

Don't have the people that you are working on repeat after you anything that you're doing. This raises their brainwaves to Beta; you do not want them to raise their brainwaves, you want them to lie or sit peacefully and quietly. When you work on them, when you touch them, it shifts their brainwaves to Theta. Theta is the key here.

In a class setting I go through the command process aloud and then as a thought form in silence and put my brainwaves back in Theta. Then I imagine going down into the client's space to observe my students work. *What is being done is happening in a fraction of a second, but you must be able to hold the Theta wave for that time.* So do not talk, just watch and listen, and you will witness the most amazing things.

THE STRUCTURE

The structure of the reading is simple:

- Begin at the heart chakra.
- Send your energy down to Mother Earth.
- Bring your energy back up into your body to open the chakras and create *kundalini*.
- Send your energy up and out of your crown chakra.
- Go through all the planes of existence, using the road map to All That Is.
- Make the connection to the Seventh Plane of Existence and the Creator of All That Is.
- Make the command to witness the reading.
- Go into the person's space.
- Witness the reading.
- Once finished, bring your energy back, rinse yourself off, ground yourself to the Earth and bring your energy back up into your body.

THE RINSING

After completing a reading or healing, it is important to visualize rinsing your consciousness to avoid leftover aches and pains or emotional baggage you may have picked up as a memory from the other person.

You can do this in one of two ways: the first is to rinse off in white light or clear water as you come back into your space with your consciousness; the second is to go back up to the Seventh Plane of Existence to rinse off. Once you have connected to the Seventh Plane your consciousness will be purified and you can open your eyes in peace. This is the *spiritual cleansing* and separation for the process.

THE GROUNDING

The definition of *grounding* is 'bringing all of our consciousness into our own space and body using the Earth'. As you bring your consciousness back into your own space, it is important that you follow these steps to 'ground' yourself correctly:

1. Visualize your energy going down into the Earth.
2. Visualize the energy coming back up through your feet, up through your body, to your crown.

Grounding in this manner will keep you from gaining excess weight, keep your energy centres open and allow the *kundalini* to open gently.

THE ENERGY BREAK

To create *physical cleansing* we use the energy break. This is a form of protection to ensure that all energetic influences such as negative feelings, emotions or other vibrations from the reading are separated from the practitioner.

THE ENERGY BREAK

1. Put your right hand and left hand palm to palm, fingers touching, wrists and elbows out to the side. The back of your right hand will be facing your chest and the back of your left hand will be facing outward. Rub your palms together. Pull your right hand back to your chest and extend the left hand away from your body toward your client. This will take care of the energy that is left over.

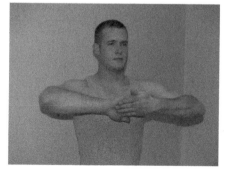

2. When you have finished making the break from the person, bring your right hand straight up in a knife position and move your hand up and down in front of your chest, making a slicing motion down toward your solar plexus.

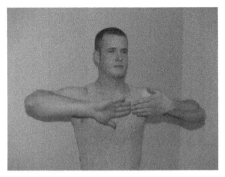

This last act aligns your polarity and, in essence, 'zips' you up again and closes your auric field. This field or bubble around you is your protection from outside influences. It is like a spiritual 'skin'. It is a field of electromagnetic energy that in most people reaches three feet up and six feet out. It has been said that the aura of the Buddha reached out for miles around him.

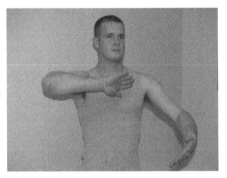

Once you have used the belief work you will no longer need to worry about rips or openings in your aura because your aura will radiate outward. Like a small sun, you will shine with your connection to the Creator.

As your understanding of ThetaHealing develops, more will be revealed to make this process even more effective.

THE READING WITH A CLIENT

Here is how to conduct a reading with a client. It is important that you go through the steps in the proper order.

THE READING

1. Seat yourself in a chair directly across from the person who is going to be receiving the reading.

2. Place your hands, palms up, on the bottom of the hands of the person, whose hands are palms down, and hold their hands in yours. (It doesn't really matter how you hold their hands.)

3. Centre yourself in your heart and visualize yourself going down into Mother Earth, which is part of All That Is.

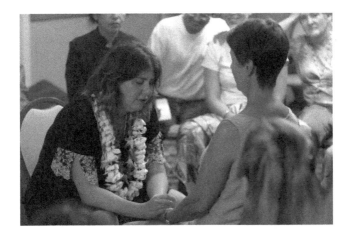

4. Visualize bringing up energy through your feet, opening up all of your chakras as you go. Go up out of your crown chakra in a beautiful ball of light out to the universe.

5. Go beyond the universe, past the white lights, past the dark light, past the white light, past the jelly-like substance that is the Laws, into a pearly iridescent white light, into the Seventh Plane of Existence.

6. Make the command and say silently, *'Creator of All That Is, a reading is commanded for [person's name].'*

7. You then say, *'Thank you.'* This is very important because when you say 'Thank you' your subconscious thinks it is already done. More importantly, you are connecting and expressing gratitude to the most important being in the universe: the Creator.

8. Now firmly state, *'It is done. It is done. It is done.'* This tells your subconscious, conscious and higher self that this action has been completed.

9. At this point (remember you are still imagining yourself above your space), imagine yourself going into the other person's body, through the top of their head (through their crown chakra), to turn on a light.

10. The reason for turning on the light when you begin doing readings is to train your mind. This is like training yourself to ride a bicycle. The first thing that happens when you turn on the light is the brain lights up – if everything is alright in that part of the body. If any part of the body does not light up as you are going through, then there is a problem in that area.

11. You then proceed to the neck. If their neck doesn't light up, then ask the person if their neck hurts. Most of the time, they will tell you that they have a whiplash injury, or they have neck pain, or you'll discover that there is a problem with their thyroid. Then proceed down through the chest. If that area lights up, go down

to their stomach. As you imagine going down through their body, inform them of any area that does not light up. Remember, every time you speak to them, your brainwaves return to Beta. However, you can easily return to Theta because you are teaching the mind to go from Beta to Alpha to Theta on command. Continue all the way down through the body.

12. When you have finished scanning their body, imagine yourself lifting up out of their space and rinsing yourself off with a stream of water. (This can be a mountain stream or a waterfall, whatever you want to imagine). Imagine your energy coming back into your space and going into the Earth. Pull the Earth energy up through all your chakras to your crown chakra. Make an energy break.

Training your mind to do a reading is exciting. It takes more than one attempt for your subconscious to 'get it', but with each reading you will reach a deeper Theta state and the details you get will be more specific. Usually when people have difficulties with readings, they are simply trying too hard, making it difficult to learn. Have faith and do a reading with joy in your heart, and it will become easy.

You might ask, 'What if I don't know anything about the body?' I suggest that you get a well-illustrated anatomy book and study it so that you can recognize the organs you are seeing. Certain things will show up in the body that you are unfamiliar with and in the beginning you aren't going to be an expert. But with time and practice you will learn.

THE PRINCIPLES OF THE READING

Θ *Throughout this book, each section will have its own set of principles or guidelines to go by when using the work.*

TALK TO THE BODY

This is an extremely powerful technique. It can be used to communicate with the body. The body communicates back to you as you are doing a reading. Cell talks to cell, and every time you appropriately touch another person's body, your body automatically communicates with their body. For instance, while working with a woman, stop at her reproductive organs and ask the body how many children it has 'housed'. The body will immediately tell you how many pregnancies it has experienced, as well as how many children are held within the heart waiting to be born. The Theta state allows you to hear what the body is saying.

One of the best experiences of the body scan is to do a reading on a pregnant woman. When you see a foetus kick and move in the uterus, you will be astounded. In fact, when you go into an expectant mother's body and view the foetus, look for the baby's genitalia to tell if it is a boy or a girl.

If you have *any* questions while you are in the body, ask the Creator. If someone is ill, ask the Creator to show you the cause. Always be precise in what you ask the Creator, because the answer will be very specific. The Creator is very direct and never makes things more complicated than they need to be.

THE HEART CHAKRA

Each time a ThetaHealer™ goes into a person's space in a reading, a person experiences having their heart chakra touched. This feeling may be unfamiliar to them. They can become confused and mistake these feelings for romantic love toward the practitioner. The practitioner must be very careful to clarify to the client that the feelings they are experiencing are caused by the reading and are only temporary. You must clarify these facts to the people that you work with.

Also, what is said in the process of a reading should be kept in the strictest confidence. *It is imperative to keep your own opinions and feelings out of the reading.* Make sure it is done through the Creator of All That Is.

THE EXCHANGE OF ENERGY

There should be an exchange of energy between the practitioner and client, whether it is money, a crystal or even a hug. The reason for this is that an exchange of energy allows the superconscious of both the practitioner and the client to recognize that something solid and physical has taken place, thereby permitting healing to take place.

THE THETA SLEEP CYCLE

When you are in Theta and use the Theta wave extensively for healings or readings, your physical body will believe that it is in a sleep cycle. You may need to push yourself to do more physical exercise to balance out the body processes.

THOUGHTS HAVE SUBSTANCE

As you begin to use Theta, as already mentioned, you should be much more careful with your thoughts. This is important because Theta opens new doorways in the mind. Your thoughts will have real substance as never before.

REMOTE VIEWING

Through the Theta technique we are able to send our consciousness through space and time to 'read' a person intuitively anywhere on the planet. This procedure also shows us that we do not have to physically touch a person to facilitate a reading.

Ask the person where they are in the world so that you know where to send your consciousness in your command process. You can visualize your consciousness travelling to the person and entering their space. This might take up to four seconds.

ETHICS IN THE READING

It is very important for the reader not to attempt to take charge of another person's life. A person's freedom of choice should never be altered or changed. If I tell a person that they will find money lying on the pavement, then they may look until they find money lying on the pavement. So it is very important that the subconscious mind of a client is not led into something that you've worked to create for them.

When you go in and do a reading on a person, you are seeing what that person's life is, not what is right for you. You should avoid interjecting your morals, your ethics or your opinions into a reading. For some people it is a definite sin to have more than one lover, for example, while for others it is an absolute part of life to have more than one person to love. Each person is an individual being living their own individual life. Everyone has different feelings and has been brought up with a different concept of what is right and wrong for them. So you should avoid telling people having a reading what is right or wrong for them to do. You may offer them your opinion about what you would do if you were in their shoes, but you should not make a decision for them. You are only to tell them what you see and give them your unbiased opinion.

Also, avoid instilling anything concerning your own life into the reading. What is going on in your life should never have anything to do with the individual being worked on. A false concept that has been widely spread is that the people you come into contact with mirror you. It is true that people can reflect certain things in your life and you can learn from these things, but no person is an absolute mirror of anyone else.

In short, the reading is sacred and is focused on the client. Therefore, if you ask questions pertaining to them, in response you will get answers pertaining to them.

6

OPENING THE PSYCHIC CENTRES THROUGH THE CHAKRAS

As your psychic abilities develop, strange things may happen. Electrical devices may short circuit, radios may turn on and off, lights may flash and you may contact 'outside' information. If this happens, you may be psychically off-balance. To alleviate this problem, keep yourself centred so that 'loose' energy does not leak out of you. Command that your psychic centres be in balance. Retaining psychic balance is as important as keeping the physical body in balance. The opening of the chakras creates this balance on all levels of our being.

OPENING THE CHAKRAS

Within the chakras the psychic senses lie waiting to blossom. They could be likened to the fragrance of the opening flower of the chakra. As a practitioner of ThetaHealing, you may find some individuals (or yourself) will have one or more of the chakras closed. If this is the case, the person (or you) will have a difficult time with readings, healings, visualizing, etc.

In some instances the crown chakra can be closed. The clairvoyant or third eye chakra might have a 'web or mesh' lying over the top of it, making it difficult or even impossible for the person to be intuitive. Don't concern yourself with where this web or mesh comes from. Simply go up and connect to God to command that it be removed and sent to God's light, never to return.

The process of opening the chakras is designed as a means of opening the psychic centres through the chakras. It is best to proceed slowly. Sensory and psychic overload are real things, so be careful of *too much too soon*. In the process of accelerating the psychic abilities, specifically ask for only as much as is for the 'highest and best' at any given time.

THE PROCESS OF OPENING THE CHAKRAS

When Working on Another Person

Go up and make the command: *'Creator of All That Is, it is commanded that this person's chakras be opened in the highest and best way. Thank you! It is done. It is done. It is done.'*

Beginning at the crown chakra, keep your hand six inches (15 cm) from the body. With a clockwise turning of the hand, visualize the opening of each chakra blossoming with the motion of the hand. You may feel the energy of the chakra in your hand as it opens. Continue until all seven chakras are open.

When Working on Yourself

Go up and make the command: *'Creator of All That Is, it is commanded that my chakras be opened in the highest and best way. Thank you! It is done. It is done. It is done.'*

Now, whether working on yourself or another person, visualize each chakra opened 'as is for the highest and best at this time', beginning at the base chakra:

- **The base chakra**
  This chakra is the support system of all the other chakras. It deals with abundance. It is what grounds us to the world around us. The Sanskrit word for it is *Muladhara*. It is the seat of *kundalini*.

- **The sacral chakra**
  This deals with sexual energy and abundance. It is associated with the qualities of movement and the flow of energy. The Sanskrit for it is *Svadistanna*.

- **The solar plexus chakra**
  This is where your empathic psychic senses are – your 'gut' feeling. The Sanskrit word for it is *Manipura*.

- **The heart chakra**
  This chakra deals with balancing emotional levels. The Sanskrit word for it is *Anahatha*.

- **The throat chakra**
  This is concerned with communication, inner identity and telepathy. It is used to give divine information. The Sanskrit word for it is *Visshuda*.

- **The third eye**

  This is the chakra that enables you to see intuitively. It is concerned with clairvoyance, intellect, belief, understanding and the analysis of reality. In Sanskrit it is called *Ajna*.

- **The crown chakra**

  This is the prophetic chakra. In Sanskrit it is called *Sahasrara*. It keeps us in constant touch with the outer universe and the subtle dimensions of spiritual energy. This chakra is connected to the whole of creation. As the base chakra connects us firmly and safely to the Earth, so the crown chakra opens us to the universal energy of the Creator of All That Is.

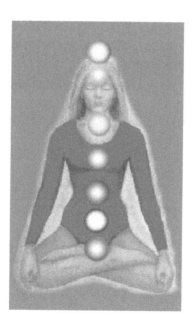

OPENING THE PSYCHIC CENTRES

The psychic centres will only open up as much as they should at any one time. Use the following process to open the psychic centres of a person by activating the chakras:

THE PROCESS OF OPENING THE PSYCHIC CENTRES

1. Centre yourself in your heart and visualize yourself going down into Mother Earth, which is part of All That Is.

2. Visualize bringing up the Earth energy through your feet, opening up all of your chakras as you go. Continue going up out of your crown chakra in a beautiful ball of light out to the universe.

3. Go beyond the universe, past the white lights, past the dark light, past the white light, past the jelly-like substance that is the Laws, into a pearly iridescent white light, into the Seventh Plane of Existence.

4. Make the command: *'Creator of All That Is, it is commanded to open [person's name]'s psychic senses in the highest and best way. Thank you! It is done. It is done. It is done.'*

5. Move your consciousness over to their space.

6. While connected to the Creator, begin with the crown chakra. Keep your hand six inches (15 cm) from the body. With a clockwise turning of the hand, visualize the opening of each chakra blossoming with the motion of the hand. In this way, open each of the seven chakras. Use the feeling in your hands to gauge the senses being opened properly.

7. As soon as you envision the process as finished, rinse yourself off. Put yourself back into your space, ground to the Earth, draw Earth energy up to your crown and make an energy break.

7

THETAHEALING

Although healings and readings are different, the two aspects will eventually blend together once you are familiar with all the branches of the ThetaHealing tree.

In one of the first instances of instantaneous healing, I witnessed the healing of a horse's broken leg. Incidents like this gave me the encouragement to continue experimenting on different infirmities. I found that ThetaHealing could be used to heal illnesses such as cancer, as in this testimonial from Sally that demonstrates the grace of the Creator of All That Is:

My name is Sally. In June 2001, I was diagnosed with malignant melanoma arising from a mole on the back of my head. This diagnosis was devastating, because melanoma does not have any effective treatment and is usually terminal.

After I had had surgery, several consultations with doctors and several pathology reviews, lesions were discovered in my brain on 11 September 2001. This news was devastating, because there is no treatment for melanoma malignancy that has spread to the brain. Usually the life expectancy is four to six months and can be as short as four weeks.

It was after this news that I became acquainted with Vianna. A family friend had heard of her success in helping people with serious medical problems and gave us the information we needed to find her.

Vianna was absolutely wonderful from the start. Even with a heavy schedule, she was able to arrange an 'emergency' session with me. During this session, she removed the brain lesions. Subsequent brain MRIs have shown they have gone. At a later time, she cleaned my blood, and a special test from the John Wayne Cancer Institute has verified that there are no melanoma cells in my blood. This essentially means that I am now clear of any cancer.

The healing, while miraculous, wasn't the only thing that was so very impressive about Vianna. She told me on my first visit that I had 'pins' in some old root canals that would give me trouble. Two months later, a massive infection was discovered that had resulted from the breakdown of the silver pins inserted during a root canal years ago. Also, after I was subjected to whole-brain radiation, I lost my sense of taste, which is a common side-effect of this treatment. In a session with Vianna, I mentioned this to her and she made adjustments to the radiation effects and that night I was able to taste again.

Vianna has always treated my husband and me with the utmost respect and friendliness. She has made room to see me when her schedule has been completely booked. She is a sincere, compassionate person that takes her healing powers in her stride. She gives the credit to God and declares that she is only the messenger. Her message to me has been one of life and hope. None of the doctors has been able to explain the changes that took place in me and they are all completely amazed that this terminal disease has simply disappeared. I know the reason and now the rest of the world can share in my knowledge. Vianna is truly a miracle-maker.

This was an excellent example of a person who had no subconscious programmes blocking the healing process. Due to her psychological make-up, Sally was ready to accept instant healing, just as I was ready to witness it done.

When I was doing the body scan, I was told that she had developed the melanoma from working at a chemical plant. I had to jog her memory for the validation that I was right, but then Sally thought back and told me that some years before she had worked in a chemical plant. This told me that the cause was environmental, due to radiation or chemicals, and I felt certain that she could be healed without reprogramming her belief systems.

When the healing happened, I witnessed the Creator pull the lesions out of her brain. It was an instantaneous healing and I could feel her body shift and heal with the Creator's Love. This energy flashed back into my space, came out of me and went back into both of us. I knew that she was instantly healed.

Now I will show you the process of healing step by step.

Θ *The Creator of All That Is is the healer and you are just the observer watching it happen.*

THE PRINCIPLES OF HEALING

This basic healing technique can be utilized on children who have hurt themselves and need immediate attention. It is wonderful to use on your family for any given situation. It is wonderful to take away a headache, to remove back pain and to command all pain to be gone. This healing technique will change your life.

VERBAL CONSENT

The question often arises as to what maladies you can heal without a person's verbal consent.

If the person being worked on is unconscious or is in an emergency state, you can ask their higher self for permission to work on them.

There are other healing techniques in this book that deal with chromosomal changes, DNA or subconscious programming. These techniques require the verbal consent of the person being worked on. This must be respected.

However, you can send unconditional love to a person at any time. Which brings us to…

UNCONDITIONAL LOVE

In order to make a molecular change in the body, one must have energy. This is a fact that goes all the way down to the smallest particle, the atom. In order for a molecule to form, it must have energy to put together the atoms that make it what it is. Knowing that it is energy that makes changes on a molecular level, there must be energy available to create this or any change.

So, in order for a cell to change and heal in the body it must have the energy to do so. The body has two ways of forming this energy: heat and enzymes. Any change in the body is created by heat and enzymes, unless the change is made through the Creator of All That Is.

When you go up to the Creator of All That Is for a healing, you reach up and grab the energy of *unconditional love* and put it in the body. This enables the body to have the energy it needs to make changes. Just commanding the body to heal on its own forces it to use its own mechanics for the energy, and these resources are generally not enough. For instance, if you command a bone to heal without extra energy, it will strip calcium from the surrounding resources of the body to comply with the command.

You may ask, 'How much of this energy do I use?' It only takes one atom of unconditional love to make any change in the body. For instance, when you make the command, *'Creator of All That Is, a change is commanded in this body,'* you will automatically see energy coming into the body to make the change.

In the beginners' classes we teach people a step-by-step process to visualize 'going up' and gathering the love. But as the brain gets used to what it is supposed to be visualizing, the process will happen automatically. In the end it is your ability to *witness* that brings the healing into the *now*. The Creator does the healing; you witness it. There is a law in physics that says nothing exists unless it is witnessed.

BLOCKING BELIEFS

Many people are ready for instantaneous healing on their body. If the body does not receive instantaneous healing when given the command, there is a subconscious programme blocking it. This programme must be found and changed. As long as the healer keeps themselves from becoming discouraged, the Creator will assist them to find that feeling, emotion or belief by using the Creator's wisdom or the wisdom of the person. The mind, body and spirit of a person have a memory like a computer and if you know the right questions to ask, these aspects of the person will tell you what needs to be released and replaced, or what feeling is missing.

It is possible, however, that the healer will misinterpret these messages and become discouraged. Or perhaps the feeling of discouragement is not the healer's, but is projected from the person being healed. Perhaps that person does not know how to live without being discouraged and therefore has lost hope.

It is my conviction that there are only a few feelings, emotions and beliefs for every specific healing. It is my understanding that disease is caused by having certain belief programmes over a long period of time. Once these beliefs are cleared, the disease leaves. Clearing it is simple, since it is designed to get your attention to tell you that something is out of synchronicity with the body, out of focus or out of balance. You simply rebalance it.

COMMUNICATION WITH THE CREATOR

It is also my conviction that ThetaHealing is not just clearing illness; it is also a way for humankind to communicate with the Creator of All That Is. The goal is to clear the body, mind and soul of enough burdening beliefs so that we can have pure and unadulterated communication with the Creator.

If you imagine ascending high above your body, you will be gathering the love of All That Is and will be assisted by that love in doing your healings. Once you connect to the All That Is energy of the Creator, you go through what is called the electromagnetic field of the Earth. When you go beyond this field, you come to a place that is past the Laws of Karma, past the areas that block you from 'becoming', into an area of unconditional love. Always bring the essence of this love into the healing. Healing is accomplished from a place of unconditional love! Never forget this undeniable fact. Healing is not done to prove a point or to demonstrate your ability to heal.

ATTACHMENT

Expect that the person will heal, but do not be attached to the outcome. The Creator of All That Is is the healer. So give up the outcome to the Creative Force. Say to your client, 'The Creator of All That Is is the healer. Let's see what happens.'

If you don't achieve the results you want, it indicates that there is belief work to be done.

THE WITNESS AND INTENTION

Witnessing the healing being done is a very important part of the process. Going up and commanding it to be done is one thing, watching it being done is another. Only after you have witnessed the healing process is it done.

I have many people tell me that as long as the healer *intends* to do it, it is done. But there is a big difference between intending to do something and doing it. I can intend to pick up my keys all day long and I can intend to be helpful to my husband. It doesn't mean that I actually have walked over and picked up my keys, nor does it mean that I have necessarily done anything to help my husband. When you go into the body, you must watch the process that you have commanded being done until it is finished. You are there to witness it in action. Without action, nothing happens. There is a distinct difference between thinking about doing something, procrastinating and actually doing it, both physically and metaphysically.

It is said that 'the road to hell is paved with good intentions', but the bad reputation of intentions is not entirely deserved. Science shows that intentions are somewhat related to later behaviour, but only modestly. Good intentions account for only about 20 to 30 per cent of the variance in the desired behaviour. Of course, strong intentions have more influence than weak intentions, but both strong and weak often fail. 'Intention' alone will not have the same effect as making the process a reality by properly witnessing the co-creative energy in the body of your client or in your own body, depending on the situation. ThetaHealing is centred on going beyond the intentions of the ego in the conscious mind to being the witness to the healing.

When a healing is witnessed or observed, it is brought into this reality through genesis by observation.

GENESIS BY OBSERVATION

In 2002, John Wheeler, a colleague of scientists such as Albert Einstein and Niels Bohr, and the man who coined the term 'black hole', asked the question, 'How come existence?' There may come a time when quantum physics may be able to prove that the act of observation changes our reality.

To test this theory, scientists created an experiment. Light was shone through two parallel slits and hit a strip of photographic paper. The experiment was done in two ways, both achieving different results. First, with photon detectors right beside each slit, physicists observed each photon as it passed through one slit or the other. The photons, in other words, acted like particles.

In the second way, the photon detectors were removed but otherwise the experiment was conducted in exactly the same fashion. However, this time the photosensitive paper showed that, instead of acting like a particle, the light acted like a wave.

We know that light has a dual nature of both particle and wave, but it seems that the mere *act of observation* influences which way it acts.

This 'reaction to observation' works on a universal scale as well. This experiment has been conducted using light that has been flung at the Earth from across the galaxy and the results were the same: the light reacted differently based on whether or not it was being observed. This means that our observations now seem to affect light waves/particles that were created millions or even billions of years before we were born. It appears that thought changes even our past or, as John Wheeler says, 'Information may not be just what we learn about the world, it may be what *makes* the world.'

Looking at how this pertains to the Theta technique, we see the aetheric pathway that is created between the healer and client and the Creative Force as a small 'wormhole'. In space and time, this wormhole permits us to cross dimensions to conduct healings and readings without the interference of time or other factors, in addition to maintaining an opening to the Creative Force so that we might utilize this energy.

In quantum mechanics, the act of observation affects the result. ThetaHealing is the act of observation. The Theta technique is quantum mechanics, and the art of visualization must be learned to make co-creation possible. This is why the *witnessing* of the healing is so important. When the healer witnesses the healing being done, it is brought into this reality.

The best way to step into the creative energy is to make the *command* to the Creator of All That Is. This tells the subconscious mind that it will be *done*. Using the word 'command' or a commanding energy will place the subconscious in a position where it cannot interfere.

ACCEPTANCE

Accept the healing as *real*. The healing energy of the Creator may bring it about so quickly that it is done before you can actually visualize it. If this occurs, command a slow-motion replay so that you are able to witness it and accept it.

A DOUBLE-EDGED SWORD

Visualization is a double-edged sword: on one side, we have the witnessing of healing as *done*, on the other side the healer can actually see a cut, burn or break with the physical eyes. When we physically 'see' a challenge to be healed, the very act of looking at the affliction brings it into reality in the mind of the practitioner. It is best when doing a healing on an open sore or wound to keep it covered as the healing is done and not to look at it. It is best to see it only with the eyes of God until you are used to instant healing.

REMOTE HEALING

As with a reading or body scan, the co-creative process of the ThetaHealing enables us to work with a client anyhere on Earth. Once a connection has been made, the reader sends their consciousness across the vast distances to enter the space of the client as if the two people were in the same room.

FEAR, DOUBT AND DISBELIEF

Fear, doubt and disbelief are the most powerful blocks to any intuitive healing. You can influence the reading by your own beliefs and fears, so if you begin to have any doubts during a reading or healing, or if you feel disconnected from the co-creative process, get out of the person's space, wash off and rest for a while, then begin the process again. You should also use the ThetaHealing belief work on yourself to get crystal clear to do the best healing possible.

You can tell that your beliefs are interfering with the reading if you have any excessive emotional reaction before, after or during it. Bear in mind, too, that the client themselves may have beliefs that keep the disease in place or block the healing from entering their space.

JOY, HAPPINESS AND LOVE

The essence of joy, happiness and love generates the healing energy used in co-creating a healing or reading. So that you can create happiness and joy in the healing, you must keep your personal affairs separate from your energy work.

It is also important to have a degree of unconditional love for people. You should genuinely care for people, because if you don't, you may find this line of work difficult.

ENVIRONMENTAL ILLNESSES

Environmental illnesses can be healed instantly; however, if the person is continually exposed to the same environmental factor, it can re-create the illness. The toxins will simply reinstate the sickness. It's suggested that to *stay* healed the person changes their lifestyle and environment and follows the healing up with belief work.

YOU ARE NEVER ALONE

You are never alone when you do a reading. You can go up and ask for help anytime, anywhere, under any circumstances.

You are never alone when you do a healing, because *you* are not doing the healing, the Creator is. This is a very important fact to remember.

BE SPECIFIC

Make your command specific enough to accomplish your goals. Once you know exactly what it is that you are going to witness in the healing, the changes can happen. The key to a good healing is to know exactly *what* you are healing.

Also, always take a moment to quiet yourself, and always make certain that when you go up and command the Creator to do whatever is needed that you remain in the person's space until you are sure that it is completed.

TIME ENOUGH TO HEAL

When in the co-creative process of ThetaHealing, *time* does not exist. It slows to a crawl or stops completely during the period when the healing is being done. This occurs because the incredible amount of work that is happening has to have time to finish without causing any difficulties on the physical, mental or spiritual levels.

You must realize that once the command is made and your mind witnesses and accepts the healing, it has already been accomplished outside the present time and reality. Being the witness brings it into this time and reality, allowing it to truly materialize and take form in the physical world.

This aspect of time is true of all the techniques of ThetaHealing.

SELF-HEALING

There is no reason why you cannot heal yourself as you would another person.

You use the healing technique on yourself in the same way as with a client by bringing the Creator into your body and witnessing the healing. This is the process that I used on my leg all those years ago and have used numerous times since for healing myself.

IN THETAHEALING, AVOID...

- Commanding all bacteria to be gone from the body, since many of the body's processes rely on bacteria to function.
- Commanding all *Candida* to be gone from the body since many of the body's processes rely on some *Candida* to function.
- Commanding all heavy metals to be gone from the body because the body is comprised of many different kinds of heavy metals, such as calcium and zinc.
- Commanding that vital minerals and vitamins be created from the Creator. Without practice, the body does not understand how to assimilate minerals and vitamins in this way.
- Commanding the body to go back to its perfect blueprint. The body is given a genetic programme from the moment of conception that tells itself that it is perfect. If there is a disease in the body, it perceives it as perfect. The body has the perfect diabetes, the perfect multiple sclerosis, and so on. Everything is perfect in its universe, therefore the subconscious will not understand this command.
- Avoid the presumption that, as the practitioner, you are the one doing the healing. It is *God* that is the healer, not you. It is best to always ask God to 'heal this' in the '*highest and best way*' and to '*show me*'.

Θ *Using the statement* 'in the highest and best way' *in a command is extremely important. This is stating that the Creator will know what is best for the person and the healer is detached from their ego long enough for the process to finish. It also detaches the healing from the influences of this plane.*

The words 'show me' *signal to the Creator that the healer will be the witness.*

HEALING

Healing may be instant or it may take several minutes. Stay focused and do not permit your mind to wander.

THE HEALING TECHNIQUE

1. Ask the client for permission.

Θ *Permission is important since it brings the client into the reality of the healing. Consent from the client will give their body permission to heal.*

2. Centre yourself in your heart and visualize going down into Mother Earth, which is part of All That Is.

3. Visualize bringing up the Earth energy through your feet, opening each chakra to the crown chakra. In a beautiful ball of light, go out to the universe.

4. Go beyond the universe, past the white lights, past the dark light, past the white light, past the jelly-like substance that is the Laws, into a pearly iridescent white light, into the Seventh Plane of Existence.

5. Go up and connect to the Creator and make the command: *'Creator of All That Is, it is commanded that this ailment be changed in [person's name] to perfect health in the highest and best way. Show me. Thank you! It is done. It is done. It is done.'*

   For example, this is the wording used to heal a person with a broken bone: *'Creator of All That Is, it is commanded that this bone become whole. Thank you! It is done. It is done. It is done.'*

6. Go into the person's space and permit the Creator to take you to the place in the body that needs to be healed.

7. Stay in the challenged area and witness as the Creator heals the person.

8. Stay there until the healing energy is finished.

Θ *It is important that you draw the energy required for the healing from the Creator, not from your own energy. This is done by commanding that it is the Creator that does the healing. You may also use the same forces to replenish your own energies after a healing.*

9. After you have witnessed the healing, go back up, rinse yourself off, put yourself back in your own space, ground yourself and make an energy break.

How effective is such healing? We have actually healed broken bones in class.

CLEARING RADIATION

This technique came from witnessing what the Creator did when brain tumours were released that were caused by too much radiation. This is the process that I witnessed when the Creator healed Sally and others.

In our industrial society we are subjected to an incredible amount of radiation from the technological wonders of the modern world. A while ago I began to notice that the cause of some cancers was radiation. So then I began to use this technique to release the day-to-day radiation of mobile phones, computers, fluorescent lights and other electrical equipment.

RELEASING RADIATION

1. Centre yourself in your heart and visualize going down into Mother Earth, which is a part of All That Is.

2. Visualize bringing up energy through your feet, opening each chakra to the crown chakra. In a beautiful ball of light, go out to the universe.

3. Go beyond the universe, past the white lights, past the dark light, past the white light, past the jelly-like substance that is the Laws, into a pearly iridescent white light, into the Seventh Plane of Existence.

4. Make the command: *'Creator of All That Is, it is commanded that all radiation that does not serve [person's name] be pulled, changed and sent to God's light. Thank you! It is done. It is done. It is done.'*

5. Witness the radiation being pulled and sent to God's light.

6. As soon as the process is finished, rinse yourself off and put yourself back into your space. Go into the Earth, pull the Earth energy up through all your chakras to your crown chakra and make an energy break.

NB Since radiation is not a substance that should be in the body, it is not necessary to replace it with anything.

8

GROUP HEALING

Many years ago, when I was teaching classes in Idaho, I was guided to teach my first group healing. Several people had the idea that the more people that were involved in a healing, the better the outcome would be. So we gathered together as a group to work on a person.

A man named Lyle was the first participant. He had injured his back at work and was in constant pain from it. I persuaded him to get onto the massage table for a group healing.

We all stood around in a circle and went up and worked on him separately while he lay on the table and waited quietly. When we had finished, he tried to get up. He could hardly move; in fact the pain was worse. This was when we realized that the Theta technique was so powerful that it could actually bring about havoc rather than peace and relief when group healing was done incorrectly.

Going up to God, I checked to see what had happened. I was shown that one person had pulled the muscles one way, while another person pulled the bones another way. I could see that one healer had pulled his back in one direction and another healer had pulled his back in another direction. So I realized that if more than one person goes up and does a healing, everyone is witnessing something different, particularly if they are forcing the healing.

Lyle slowly got up from the table and tried to escape from the clutches of the healers. It took some persuasion on my part before he reluctantly got back onto the table for another healing.

When we settled him down I gathered the group around me and this time I asked the Creator for instructions. I was told to have only one person as the practitioner. The others were to stand around the table and send their love out to a certain place so that the practitioner could reach out and grab this extra love and pull it down into the person.

Following these instructions, I went up above myself to the All That Is energy and all those who were standing around the table sent their love up to me. Group healing was born. I went up and gathered the love and brought it down into Lyle and witnessed it being sent into every cell of his body. The Creator corrected the back problem and this time Lyle stood up able to move comfortably, feeling no pain.

When the healing was finished I asked him how he felt. He said, 'Vianna, the pain has all gone, but don't heal it completely because I still have a settlement with the workers' insurance. If it is completely healed, I won't be able to collect my settlement money.' At last report he has never had to have surgery.

We also used this technique on a woman who had been in a wheelchair for 18 years. We went up and sent unconditional love to every cell in her body. When we had finished, she could feel her feet. The second time we worked on her, she could feel her legs. Did she come back for more healings? No, she did not. She was receiving disability benefits and was absolutely terrified that if we continued to work with her, she might actually get to the point where she could walk again and would lose her benefits.

You cannot heal someone who does not want to be healed. It is their choice and their right to make that choice. You must respect this.

Now, having witnessed hundreds of group healings, I can testify they are a wonderful way for a group of people to bond in unconditional love and perform phenomenal healing. Over the years I have learned a great deal about group healings and their amazing effects.

THE PRINCIPLES OF GROUP HEALING

Group healing trains people to hold their concentration in a Theta state and helps with visualization skills. It enables people to gather universal energy for co-creational healing and to witness healing energy in the body.

It also allows the client to feel what it's like to receive unconditional love – the highest vibration in the universe – and gives the members of the group the opportunity to bestow unconditional love on someone without restriction.

When a person does not feel unconditional love after their group healing, this informs you that they have the belief that they cannot accept unconditional love.

DECORATING

In group healing you learn to avoid being the director of the healing, to avoid 'decorating' the process with your ego. You discover how to simply witness a person being healed by the Creator of All That Is.

Here is the process for group healing:

THE GROUP HEALING PROCESS

Appoint one person to be the practitioner. Others in the group can stand around the person being healed, either holding hands or just sending their energy up to the Creator to hold it there for the practitioner.

The practitioner should appropriately place both hands on the person being healed.

1. **People around the circle**: Centre in your heart and visualize going down into Mother Earth, which is a part of All That Is.

2. Visualize bringing up energy through your feet, opening each chakra to the crown chakra. In a beautiful ball of light, go out to the universe.

3. Go beyond the universe, past the white lights, past the dark light, past the white light, past the jelly-like substance that is the Laws, into a pearly iridescent white light, into the Seventh Plane of Existence.

4. Send your unconditional love up to the power of the Creator and hold this unconditional love to be collected by the practitioner.

5. **Practitioner**: Go up to the Creator and make the command: *'Creator of All That Is, it is commanded that unconditional love be sent through every cell of [person's name] and that healing be done on this day. Thank you! It is done. It is done. It is done.'*

6. Collect this unconditional love and bring the energy down. Then direct the energy through every cell of the individual's body in co-created healing.

7. As soon as the process is finished, rinse yourself off and put yourself back into your space. Go into the Earth, pull Earth energy up through all your chakras to your crown chakra and make an energy break.

8. **People around the circle**: Rinse yourself off and put yourself back into your space. Go into the Earth, pull Earth energy up through all your chakras to your crown chakra and make an energy break.

9

WHY PEOPLE DO NOT HEAL

As my healing practice began to grow, I came to see that I still had much to learn. There were certain individuals who came to me that would not heal, so I asked the Creator, 'Why?'

I was given many reasons. In many of the instances, the Creator would tell me it was because of genetics. Believing this was something that I could not change or resolve, I would tell the person, 'Sorry, it's genetic.' At the time I had no idea that it was possible to intuitively heal genetic defects.

Finally, after *I* was diagnosed with what was considered to be a genetic defect, I asked the Creator how to repair this defect. The Creator answered by showing me how to change genetic defects and told me that there were 16 additional lessons to learn. I was amazed, since the information on the DNA activation in my first book, *Go Up and Seek God*, took only one lesson.

Anxiously, I waited to receive the 16 lessons. After receiving the first one, I immediately put the information to work. The results continued to improve, but I still found that there were people who could not be helped. I would go to the Creator in the middle of a healing and ask, 'Creator, what is blocking the healing?' and would hear a voice that said, 'This person believes he should be sick' or 'This person believes that he must be punished' or 'This person believes what her doctor tells her' or 'This person really wants to die.' Thinking that I had no right to change a person's beliefs, or even remotely allow myself to have such a thought, I would send the people home, telling them that they needed to work on how they felt about themselves.

Before 1999, I had used hypnosis and emotional release techniques to change subconscious thought patterns. When I used these techniques I had only been able to change a few patterns slowly, one at a time. Also, the results were not consistent enough for me to consider integrating these techniques into my everyday healing.

Then, in 1999, the Creator showed me that you could change several patterns in seconds. I found that I was able to alter belief patterns such as 'You're not smart enough', 'You're not good enough', 'Money is bad', 'Money is evil', 'I can't be psychic', 'I'm not a healer' or 'I am separate from God'. I found that this would also work on other belief systems, too, such as 'I will suffer', 'I must have this disease' or 'It is in my genes'. I found that these, in addition to other patterns, could be changed in seconds.

As I used the techniques that I had received from the Creator, I found a pattern began to form, a pattern that I believe will change the face of energy healing forever.

ILLNESS AS INDIVIDUAL STATEMENT

An important dynamic I have discovered in healing work is that every person is different and every illness is an individual statement of who that person is. Whether they have been contaminated by heavy metals, poisons or toxins, or exposed to radiation, or whether their illness has been caused by emotional problems such as anger, grief, hatred or personal tragedies, their disease is as individual as they are. Illnesses, whether physical, emotional, environmental or a combination of all three, should be treated in that manner: individually.

For example, at the time that I was healed from lymphatic cancer I was in an unsupportive and dysfunctional marriage. I felt as though I was in limbo, powerless to change situations in my life. Several individuals told me that I had created my own cancer because of my feelings. My intuition told me that this was incorrect. I was sure that my cancer had been created by mercury poisoning. I believed this to such an extent that I did many cleanses to clear out the large amount of mercury that I knew was in my system. Once I had cleaned out the mercury, I believed that I deserved an instantaneous healing. The day I commanded myself to heal with the Theta technique, my body was healed in an instant. The reason it was healed in an instant was because I believed that I didn't have to be sick and that I could get better.

What I found was that heavy metals such as mercury carried with them certain projected thought forms and beliefs that would affect the person that they resided in. Once the mercury was gone, these influences would be gone as well. My cancer was caused by the mercury and while that mercury stayed in my system I was unable to *believe* the cancer could be healed. Toxins have their own energetic influences upon the body much as emotions and belief systems do.

As a person's life unfolds, they are subjected to a vast array of feelings and emotions, many of which become belief systems. Belief systems in and of themselves can also cause people to fall ill. Hatred actually feeds cancer, and cancer grows from hatred as a means of encapsulating the hate.

As feelings and emotions become belief systems, they change and evolve. In their negative form, beliefs can have adverse effects on heart, mind, body and soul. A person's emotions and beliefs play a significant role in whether or not you can heal them. To clarify, their emotions are a large factor in whether they believe that they can be allowed to get better, or whether they should stay ill or die.

There was a time when I worked 14 hours a day doing half-hour readings and healings back to back, six days a week. I was in the rapture of Theta, in the ecstasy that can only come from a pure connection to the Creator. The healing energy of Theta took me on its wings and I watched as patterns began to emerge in the people that came to see me. After working with thousands of people, I realized that those who believed they should be sick stayed sick. This made it almost impossible to heal them and have them remain healthy. On the other end of the spectrum, I found that people who believed they *could* be healed, who believed they *should* be healed, or believed that they *deserved* to be healed, were restored to health. I have experienced this to be true in nine cases out of ten.

SOMETIMES DEATH IS THE HEALING

Another group of people that you will encounter are those who just want to die. When working with this group you will come to realize that it makes no difference whether they believe in healers or not, or whether you believe they can heal. In the end, you must respect their decision.

A female client came to me to be healed from thyroid cancer. This is a very easy cancer to treat with conventional medicine if caught in its early stages. However, this woman had let her cancer go uncontrolled, until at last it had spread throughout her whole system. When the tumour had destroyed her vocal cords and grown to the size of a grapefruit, she tried to have it removed, but it had grown too large. When she first came to see me she was very ill and I could sense that she was dying. Her husband, however, determined to save her, was trying all kinds of alternative health techniques.

Working with this lady, I decided to use Colour Light Therapy accompanied by healing. When I first began to work on her with Theta I could see that the healing was not as effective on her as it had been on other people I had treated with similar challenges. During this time I was observing which people responded and which did not, always curious to know why. I asked myself, 'What could this woman possibly be gaining from being so sick?'

When I talked to her, she explained to me that during her battle with cancer she had found that her relationship with her husband had became close for the first time in years. They had been spending time together and she expressed her joy in that time. From an observational and therapeutic perspective, it was a very enlightening situation for me. Was this why she had cancer? To be loved? Do we create situations of a negative nature to get a positive result?

After I had worked with her a couple of times, she left and did not return for four months. When she came in again, it was heartrending to see her because I could perceive that she was critically ill. It seemed that she had improved a great deal after her first two visits, so she had decided she didn't need to see me anymore, but after about a month she had begun to get very ill again.

I took her in and began to do a session with her. As I was doing the reading with her I went up and asked the Creator, 'What is going on with this person?' The Creator said, 'Vianna, this person doesn't want to be here. She doesn't want to live.' I asked her, 'Do you want to live?' She said yes, but she was very upset that her husband had been called back to work and was no longer spending time with her.

Once again I worked with her only to have her leave and not return for regular healing. Then, several weeks later, I received a telephone call from her husband. He told me that she was in hospital and it was likely that she was going to die. He asked if I would come in to see her. I said, 'Yes, of course I will.'

Upon my arrival, he asked me to please tell him what she was thinking, for she was no longer able to speak. When I went to speak to her mind I discovered that she wanted to go home. She told me that she was finished with her life and said goodbye to her husband. I told her husband what she had said and, in tears, watched her choose to leave this life to go beyond the veil.

'LET ME GO'

Another woman came to me with the challenge of breast cancer. The cancer had ravaged her body to the point that her entire breast was gone. When I sat down with her and asked her if she wanted to live, she told me, 'No.' She said that she was tired of listening to her sister and her husband fight. It seems that the sister was furious with the husband for not permitting his wife the benefit of pain relief. He felt that she needed to suffer for her sins on Earth. She told me she was tired of the pain and the hassle. She wanted to die!

I listened to her very carefully while she told me her story. I then went up and commanded her body to be relieved of pain. I also knew that she needed emotional release therapy. So I commanded to witness the Creator taking care of her and helping her in her plight. Three days later she died after having an emotional release from a very close friend of mine.

I was unable to keep her from leaving, because I knew she wanted to die, but after she had died her husband called me. He thanked me for helping his wife and easing her passing. It was a very strange experience for me.

THE DEATH SENTENCE

In another instance I watched a long-time client who became a dear friend, Mrs Crandall, suffer with colon cancer. The doctors informed her that it was likely to take her life within two weeks.

One day she came in for her usual session and I could intuitively see that she was completely rid of colon cancer. Her doctor found no trace of colon cancer either, but told her that didn't mean she didn't still have the cancer. He held fast to the earlier pronouncement of death.

After her healing, Mrs Crandall suddenly found herself looking after her daughter's seven-month-old baby. Still recovering from the devastation of cancer and weighing barely five and a half stone (80 pounds), she nevertheless raised her granddaughter. I saw her frequently, often just to talk and give her encouragement. She wrote me the following poem:

> I hope you see, you are special to me.
> My life was a soap, but you gave me hope.
> You were around, when the doctors let me down.
> You made me laugh when I wanted to cry.
> You made me realize that I don't want to die.
> You stood by me from the start.
> I just want to thank you with all of my heart.

A year and a half later, she faced an obstruction in her bowel. The doctor still thought that no matter what was done for her she was dying, but her oncologist advised her to remove the rest of her colon 'just to be sure'. I suggested that she seek a second opinion from a more reputable oncologist. Unfortunately, she allowed the rest of her colon to be removed instead of just clearing out the obstruction, which turned out not to be cancer.

After her pointless surgery and the removal of her healthy colon, her doctor told her that she was going to die and would never go home from the hospital. I remember her crying to me on the telephone, telling me that her children wanted her to die and had already divided up her estate.

She *did* make it home from the hospital, but once she was at home, her children would not allow anyone to visit her or do any healing work with her. I tried to see her, but was turned away. Her family would not let her do anything to save herself. Forced to give in to the will of others, my wonderful friend just gave up and died.

AN EMERGING PATTERN

These are some stark examples of how real belief systems are and why they should be changed. For a long time I didn't believe changing beliefs was possible unless you did lengthy reprogramming work on yourself. I knew beliefs could be changed with hypnosis, and I knew that they could be changed with goals in mind, but I didn't realize that they could be changed in 30 seconds.

In the meantime I discovered that physical illnesses were as individual as the sufferers themselves. This is the pattern that began to emerge:

- If the cause of the illness was exposure to toxins, the body simply needed to be cleaned up and healed.
- If the cause of the illness was something in the person's belief system, that belief needed to be cleaned up and healed.
- If the cause of the illness was something genetic, that too needed to be cleaned up and healed.

I came to the realization that there are many factors that cause illness. Feelings cause illness and illness causes feelings. They go hand in hand. Feelings, emotions, toxins, injuries, genes, genetic belief systems, historical belief systems and soul belief systems are all possible factors.

The first key to assisting a person is to learn what is causing the problem. To know the cause you need to go up and ask the Creator. You are never alone when you do a healing or reading. The Creator is always with you.

10

BELIEF SYSTEMS

Belief: The acceptance by the mind that something is true or real, often underpinned by an emotional or spiritual sense of certainty.

Modern science is reaching an age of enlightenment. New avenues of thought are stirring and the earlier view that the mind and the body are separate is falling away. The awareness that emotions, feelings and the power of thought have a direct bearing upon our physical health is becoming mainstream.

This has been shown in the development of psychoneuroimmunology, a scientific discipline that is focused primarily upon the central nervous systems, the neuroendocrine system and the immune system, and their interrelationships. The central nervous system is a huge collection of connections throughout the body, incorporating sympathetic and parasympathetic systems. It allows the brain to send information throughout the body using chemicals generally referred to as 'information substances'. It was once thought that the brain sent out these information substances to respond to problems in the body and that the communication was one-way. What has now become clear is that the central nervous system controls the body's defence mechanisms. Knowing this, we can comfortably assume that every thought, emotion, idea or belief has a neurochemical consequence.

The chemical messengers of the body, called neuropeptides, were at one time thought to be found only in the brain. Pioneering research by neuropharmacologist Candace Pert has now revealed that they are present on both the cell walls of the brain and in the immune system. As these complex messengers travel throughout the body they provide vital information and sometimes almost instant physical feedback. If you have ever been in a car accident you may have found yourself shivering because of the release of adrenaline. Once the danger is over you send the message to the body's receptors that all is fine and begin to calm down. This is a simple example of how quickly information can be transmitted from thought to physiology.

Research has also indicated that an inextricable chemical link exists between our emotions, including all the stress in our lives, both good and bad, and the regulatory systems of the endocrine and immune systems through the central nervous system. This emphasizes the importance of expressing our emotions both verbally and physically in an appropriate way. When strong emotions such as fear, anger or rage are not expressed in a healthy way then the body's natural response is that of the sympathetic nervous system, as demonstrated in Walter B. Cannon's research on homoeostasis and the fight or flight syndrome. Inappropriate storing of these stressful emotions produces an excess of epinephrine and this causes a chemical breakdown, resulting in the internal weakening of the immune system and an increased potential for disease.

We can safely say that thoughts, words, emotions and the physical body are all synergistically linked together. A thought is expressed in an electromagnetic brainwave that sends a message to the neuropeptides, which in turn are fired off into the central nervous system to produce the appropriate result from the human body. A belief system is a strong enough (or perhaps recurring) thought that is relayed to the neuropeptides within the message system of the body. In turn, the physical body reacts to the emotional belief systems to which it is conditioned. The key is to change the messages that are sent to the body, and to do that we have to change our *beliefs*.

HOW TO CHANGE BELIEFS

THE CONSCIOUS MIND

The conscious mind can be compared to a word processor. It is the decision-maker for our day-to-day affairs. It sends the subconscious mind programmes to perform certain tasks, observes how the subconscious programmes perform and then decides on what else needs to be done.

The conscious mind is estimated to be only 12 per cent of our mind. What it perceives as a belief isn't exactly what our subconscious believes. You may think that you have absolutely no subconscious limitations on abundance or money, for example. To the conscious mind, it doesn't make any logical sense that there would be restrictions within the subconscious, or for that matter on any other level of your being, but they may be there nevertheless.

A unique quality of the conscious mind is that it can quickly judge what is right and what is wrong, something that the subconscious doesn't do. The conscious decides what information should be kept in the brain and what should not, at least to some degree.

THE SUBCONSCIOUS MIND

The subconscious mind is like a computer's hard drive. It contains all of our memories, habits, beliefs, characteristics and self-image, and controls autonomic bodily functions. It is both the storeroom of information and the performer of tasks. It also contains 'predefined instructions' that we do not have to consciously think about, such as keeping our heart beating.

The subconscious is estimated to be 88 per cent of the mind. This means that when we recognize that one of our beliefs is negative, 12 per cent of our mind wants to change the other 88 per cent. Any decision to change is first formed in our conscious mind. This decision will in some way conflict with existing beliefs.

THE BODY

The body is like the computer hardware, set up to respond to the programming. Every second of every day our body is responding to the programming that is sent from the subconscious mind *automatically*. However, there is some evidence that the body has an intelligence of its own. In an experiment, cells that were subjected to nutrients gravitated toward the nutrition. When subjected to toxins, they retreated.

OPENING THE MIND FOR POSITIVE CHANGE

The conscious mind can program the subconscious mind for new behaviour and habits. This ability is built into us. Nobody taught us how to walk or how to talk. These accomplishments of 'self-education' were completed through an intuitive process at a very early age. Unfortunately, as we grow older, many of us get stuck in old behaviour patterns that no longer serve us, and we forget this intuitive ability of self-education.

By its nature, belief work is a means of changing behaviour. The behaviour may be physical, mental or metaphysical in nature. One of the best ways to change beliefs is through a return to innocence. When we are children our brainwave pattern is open to receiving and accepting new information. This is why the Theta state is so important, as it returns the subconscious to the frequency of growth and change. It opens the mind for positive change and returns our mentality to the purity of a child.

The reason why therapists find it so difficult to change the belief systems of a client is because they cannot directly access the subconscious mind.

Belief work is a means of doing just that: accessing the subconscious mind. But belief work takes us a step further: it gives us the ability to change beliefs that go beyond the subconscious, into the spiritual plane.

The following story is good example of how a programme is re-created and handed down from generation to generation, and how the *progression* of that programme can be broken by free will.

When I was a young girl, my mother had the old-school attitude that you should discipline your children with physical punishment. Out of all of her children, I was the only one who would run and hide. At times, I would hide under my bed to get away from her. When she told me to 'go find a switch', I would select a stick, only to break it into little pieces when she hid it for later use, rendering it unusable. I was a bit different from my siblings in that I did not blindly accept the beatings.

In time, I grew up and had my own children. Eventually my son Joshua reached a point (like all children) where he began to show defiance. One day I told him to do something and he turned to me and insolently said, 'No!' So I began to follow the programme that my mother had given me when I was a child. As she would have done, I reached over and grabbed him by the neck. But in the nick of time, I held myself back. For the first time as a young mother I began to question myself.

As my children began to explore their disciplinary boundaries, the old programme of 'go find a switch' reared its ugly head. One day all three of my children got into trouble at once and I told my precious little ones to go find a switch so that I could beat them just as my mother had taught me. When they came back, each bringing their own monstrous beating implements with them, something turned over inside me. I thought to myself, 'How could I do this to my little ones?' As they each gave me their switch, I admonished each of them in turn. If the stick was too big, I said, 'What is wrong with you? Don't you know that this will bruise you? Go outside and play!' If the stick was thin and whip-like, I said, 'What is wrong with you? Don't you know that this will raise welts on you? Go outside and play!' When I had sent each of my children away without a beating, I felt a strange sense of liberation – it felt as though something inside me had changed. In retrospect, I see that I had broken a core and possibly genetic programme that had been handed down from my mother.

For several years, the Creator had been putting together the mosaic of the belief work in my brain. As my mind was ready to accept the concept, a new branch to the sacred tree of ThetaHealing had grown. Believing that

I was ready to know how to change beliefs and that it was possible, I did what I had always done: I went to the Creator and commanded, '*Creator, how can beliefs be changed? Show me.*' I was shown that the technique that I was using for healing could also change beliefs.

I was also shown that in order for healing to happen, the person receiving the healing had to *want* to be restored to health and the person giving the healing had to *believe* it was possible. In ThetaHealng, even though it is the Creator who is doing the healing, you are the witness. If you believe that the healing is impossible, witnessing the healing will also be impossible. However, if the person doesn't want to be healed or doesn't think they can be healed, you can help them with *belief work*.

PROGRAMMES

Belief work gives us direct access to the world of our subconscious mind and a means of changing the beliefs in it. Our brain works like a biological super-computer, assessing information and responding. How we respond to an experience depends on the information that is given to the mind and how it is received and interpreted. When a belief has been accepted as real by the body, mind or soul it becomes a 'programme'.

Programmes can work to our benefit or detriment, depending on what the programme is and how we are reacting to it. Many people live most of their life with the hidden programme that they cannot succeed. Even if they are very successful for many years, they may suddenly lose everything they own or do something to defeat themselves. Without realizing that they may be sabotaging themselves, they continue the process. They do not understand that there are programmes deep within them that have been there since childhood, floating in the subconscious mind, waiting for the opportunity to be inserted into reality.

Belief work empowers people with the ability to remove these negative programmes and replace them with positive ones from the Creator of All That Is.

THE BELIEF LEVELS

There are four levels of beliefs within a person:

THE CORE BELIEF LEVEL

Core beliefs are what we are taught and accept from childhood in this life. They are beliefs that have become a part of us. They are held as energy in the frontal lobe of the brain.

THE GENETIC LEVEL

At this level, programmes are carried over from ancestors or are being added to our genes in this life. These beliefs are energies stored in the morphogenetic field around the physical DNA. This 'field' of knowledge is what tells the mechanics of the DNA what to do.

THE HISTORICAL LEVEL

This level concerns memories from past lives or deep genetic memory or collective consciousness experiences that we carry into the present. These memories are held in our auric field.

THE SOUL LEVEL

This level is all that a person is. Here the programmes are pulled off the completeness of the individual, beginning at the heart chakra, outward.

ENERGY TESTING

In order to find if a person had certain belief programmes, a simple method was developed for testing on the four levels of belief called 'muscle testing' or 'energy testing'. It originated from the conventional form of medical diagnostic kinaesiology.

Conventional kinaesiology is the scientific study of human movement. It encompasses human anatomy, physiology, neuroscience, biochemistry, biomechanics, exercise psychology and the sociology of sport. The relationship between the quality of movement and overall human health is also studied. Kinaesiological information is applied in such fields as physical therapy, occupational therapy, chiropractic, osteopathy, exercise physiology, kinaesiotherapy, massage therapy, ergonomics and athletic coaching.

Applied kinaesiology (AK) is considered a pseudoscience related to diagnostic kinaesiology. It is a method that purportedly gives feedback on the physical properties of the body. AK practitioners say that when properly applied, the outcome of an AK test, such as a muscle strength test, will determine the best form of therapy for clients. Applied kinaesiology is a form of alternative medicine, and is therefore distinct from academic kinaesiology.

THETAHEALING ENERGY TESTING

ThetaHealing uses the muscle test not to diagnose disease or study the movement of body mechanics, but to test for belief programmes within the four levels we have discussed. It is a procedure in which the practitioner is directly testing the energy field or All That Is essence of a person. This is why we call it 'energy testing'.

In belief work, the energy test is useful as a way of uncovering the client's belief programmes and where they are on the levels. It is accurate regardless of whether the person is conscious that they have the beliefs.

Energy testing allows both the practitioner and the client to experience a reaction to a stimulus – the physical and visual validation that the belief programme exists and that it has been changed. In response, they *believe* the belief programme is released and a new one is in place.

Muscle testing was the last key to unlocking belief work. There was a time when I was sceptical about it. This was because in all the sessions where I was muscle tested, the procedure was inaccurate for me. Then I met a practitioner who showed me that the body must be properly hydrated for muscle testing to work. Once the body is properly hydrated, muscle testing is a useful tool. I can assure you that through proper facilitation of energy testing your subconscious will tell you what you believe regardless of the conscious mind.

We will discuss two distinct methods for energy testing in belief work. It should be known that once the practitioner is accomplished at belief work they will not need energy testing to discover the programmes in a client. Energy testing is still useful, however, for the validation of the client.

The following pictures illustrate a weak or 'no' response and a strong or 'yes' response.

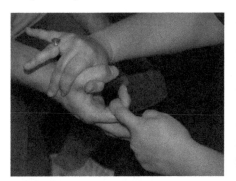 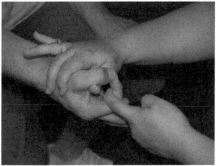

An indication of a 'no' response.   An indication of a 'yes' response.

ENERGY TESTING: METHOD ONE

Sit down opposite the client. With an up and down motion, move your hand in front of their chest, making a slicing motion downward and back up again. This will 'zip them up', pulling their electromagnetic field together so that they will energy test correctly.

1. Have the client put their thumb and either their forefinger or ring finger together in a circle. Tell them to hold their fingers together tightly.

2. Instruct them to say 'I am a man' or 'I am a woman', depending on gender, i.e. if they are a woman, prompt them to say 'I am a woman.'

3. Pull their fingers apart to gauge a 'strong' or 'weak' hold. The fingers should hold very tightly, indicating a strong, or 'yes', answer. If they come loosely apart, this indicates a weak, or 'no', answer. This indicates to the practitioner that the person is dehydrated, and testing cannot proceed with until they are hydrated:

   Give the client a glass of water, and perhaps even a tiny pinch of salt if you feel it will hydrate them faster. Salt or water will fool the body into thinking it is hydrated.

   After they have taken some of the water, have them hold the thumb and finger together tightly again and once again say 'I am a woman' or 'I am a man' as appropriate. If this time the fingers hold tightly, the practitioner knows this is a 'yes'.

   Now ask them to say 'I am a man', if a woman, or 'I am a woman', if a man. If the finger and thumb hold tightly again, indicating a 'yes' answer, this indicates that they are still dehydrated. Have them drink more water and test them again.

   Once they are holding their fingers tightly when they say they are the correct gender and they cannot do so when they say that they are the incorrect one, they are hydrated and ready to muscle test.

The practitioner needs to be observant and make sure that the client holds their fingers together firmly at all times and releases them in an unconscious manner when making the statements. Be careful that they do not try to open or close their fingers in an attempt to manipulate the procedure.

ENERGY TESTING: METHOD TWO

There is another type of muscle test that you can use when healing yourself, with someone on the telephone or even with clients that are in your presence.

1. While standing facing north, the person being tested should say, 'Yes.' Their body should lean forward for a positive answer.

2. When they say, 'No,' their body should lean backwards, indicating a negative response.

3. If their body does not lean at all, they are likely to be dehydrated.

4. If they move forward on a 'no' answer or backward on a 'yes' answer, this also indicates dehydration.

5. Once the person leans toward north for 'yes' and leans backward for 'no', they are ready to be tested for programmes.

THINGS TO NOTE WHEN ENERGY TESTING

- If the client is difficult to hydrate, have them put their hands on their kidneys (just below the ribs of the back). This will fool the body into thinking it is hydrated.
- If the person being tested spoke another language as a child, the subconscious mind may have programmes locked in place in that language. So they may not test correctly because the programme was locked in place using their native tongue. Direct them to say the programme aloud in their native tongue, or in the language that the programme was formed in. It is also necessary to say the commands with the Creator in the same native language in order to replace programmes on all four levels. Ask the client how to say the programme and use it as you would any other command.
- If someone feels uncomfortable saying 'I am a man/woman' then simply have them say 'yes' or 'no'.
- The unconscious mind does not understand words like 'don't', 'isn't', 'can't' and 'not', so you should tell the client to omit these words in their statements when in the belief work process. For example, a client should not use a statement such as 'I don't love myself' or 'I can't love myself.' To properly test for a programme, the statement should be 'I love myself.' The client will then energy test negatively or positively for this programme.
- A belief may be on only one level.
- A person might not lean or move forward or backward if they do not know what the 'feeling' is of the programme that they are testing for. It may be necessary to instil the feeling that they are unfamiliar with (*see page 98*).
- Instead of sitting directly opposite or in front of the other person, when muscle testing you should sit offset from them so as not to interfere with their auric field.
- ThetaHealing energy testing does not:
  Validate that you have reached the key belief of a 'stacked' belief system in a client (*see page 102*).
  Verify that you and the client have finished with a particular issue or with the session.
  Validate in any way the consumption or dosage of a supplement or medication.

11

How to Work on the Four Levels

You may have heard that you are what you eat. In ThetaHealing, we believe that you are what you think.

Our thoughts are created by our experiences. Our experiences in turn are created by our perceptions of the world and other people's perceptions of us. We send out signals and others perceive us through these projected thought forms. When I teach in Australia, some people think I'm from India. Some people bring me bindis to wear over my third eye, which I'm very happy to do. Is it just possible that many of them remember me from a lifetime in India, or that my vibration reminds them of it?

When I opened up my shop, people brought me so many Egyptian gifts that I made an Egyptian room. Then they brought me so many Native American gifts that I made a Native room. We are a perception of ourselves interpreted by the perceptions of other people. But what exactly is it that we believe ourselves to be?

Beliefs that have been taught in childhood and experiences that solidified in childhood can create core beliefs. The mind of a child is so delicate and perceives the parents as the first gods and goddesses in their life. Much of what is said and done to us as children is taken literally. These first imprints influence what a child will believe and won't believe. This is why we must be very careful when we talk to a child, because everything that is said is going into that child's little mind like a message from the Divine. I have often stopped to ponder all the things that could have been changed in so many lives if we had just been more careful about what we said and how we said it.

THE FOUR LEVELS

THE CORE LEVEL

Core Beliefs

Core beliefs are what we have been taught and have accepted in this lifetime from the point of conception to the present. As we exist in this space and time we are building new core beliefs all the time – even as we read and assimilate this text.

The Acceptance or Denial of a Core Belief

We always have a choice as to the programmes that we accept or deny. It is through the awareness of this ability that we attain a kind of mastery over our own destiny through the exercise of free will.

The choice to accept or deny a projected programme becomes starkly apparent when we examine how four different children react to negativity and a core belief. Each one is given a message of 'You will never amount to anything':

1. One child takes the statement literally and 'amounts to nothing', as was dictated by the programme.
2. The second child becomes an over-achiever, constantly attempting to prove the programme wrong. They never feel satisfied or good enough.
3. The third child accepts the negative programme as 'real', yet has an influential person in their life who shows them how wonderful they truly are. They believe in both programmes at the same time. (This is how a dual belief system is formed.)
4. The fourth child rejects the programme completely and follows a path of free will.

Location

The core belief level is housed as energy in the neurons at the forefront of the brain.

THE GENETIC LEVEL

Genes are the most intricate part of the body. They make up programmes to make sure that everything works. A gene is a series of nucleic acids located inside the nucleus of the cells that make up your deoxyribonucleic acid, or DNA. Your DNA consists of 23 pairs of chromosomes. Inside each of those pairs is a mechanism that runs over 100,000 functions for each strand of DNA. For every one of the 46 chromosomes there are two strands of DNA.

DNA itself is a very beautiful thing to behold in a reading. It runs everything that happens inside the body.

Over time, the cells in your body can become weak and begin to die off. DNA then takes over and gives the cells the signals that they need to re-create themselves.

The basic structure of DNA is two very long chains that run around each other, one going east and the other going west. The chain consists of four different kinds of nucleic acids in what is called the ladder. The DNA itself is compiled by what is called a shipper.

Rather than scientifically explain the functions of every particular part of the shipper and nucleic acids, suffice to say that there are over 100,000 genes located in the DNA sequence and the encodement of the double helix. DNA is so long, tied up in such a tight coil in the cells, that if you were to take it out and stretch it, it would be as tall as a man. There is an incredible amount of information encoded in each cell of your body.

Now here's the mysterious part! Around these strands is a strange field of knowledge called the morphogenetic field. This field holds genetic feelings and emotions. It is a field of knowledge that tells DNA to be DNA. It tells a baby's cells how many legs, how many feet and how many hands it's going to have.

Within this construct of DNA is genetic memory that goes back at least seven generations and in the morphogenetic field are belief systems that are holding on to information that has been stored by past generations for centuries. We're not just physical, we're mental and spiritual energy as well, and it has been found that many things that we do in our lives are not just governed by what we believe, but by what our ancestors believed also. Beliefs can be handed down from generation to generation, from one person's belief system into another person's, via the morphogenetic field.

Genetic-level programmes are those that are carried over from our ancestors or are added to our genes in this life. As with all programmes, some are to our benefit, some not.

When a Theta practitioner witnesses a genetic programme being removed and replaced, it is likely to be removed and replaced in our future, past and present energetic genetics, and those of our siblings, ancestors, parents and extended family.

Location
The genetic level is held in the centre of the brain, inside the pineal gland, as energy in the morphogenetic field around the master cell (*see page 83*). As we witness the changes occurring in the master cell, the changes are replicated in all the cells of the body.

THE HISTORY LEVEL

There are three molecules that we carry with us from life to life. When the spirit enters the body, these three molecules come to rest in three different parts of the physical body: one in the pineal gland in the brain, another in the heart and the third at the base of the spine. When *kundalini* begins to awaken, so do these molecules and the memories they carry.

It has been said that memories are carried in the subconscious mind and in the genetic or morphogenetic field, but with some memories it is difficult to identify exactly where they originate. These are called past-life memories.

Because of the highly debated issue of past-life memories and whether or not they truly come from past lives, however, it was decided to call this level the history level. On this level can be found deep genetic memories, memories of people that we have watched or been in direct contact with, and memories of other times and places.

The opening to group consciousness and the astral plane is also held on this level. Many programmes that are on this level are the result of a 'collective consciousness' due to our interconnectedness with other human thought forms. These thought forms are the result of thousands of years of human experiences, both positive and negative. As we become more intuitive, the ideas and thoughts of others can flow into our brain from the collective consciousness or even directly from other people. These ideas and thoughts affect our subconscious belief systems without us ever knowing about it.

When resolving programmes on this level, it is very important that you give all the time and attention to the process that you gave to the previous levels. The energy of this level can be seductive to the beginner. Once you connect with it, it is important to retain your grip on reality.

The history level is concerned with memories from past-life or collective consciousness experiences that we are carrying into the present. These energies must be resolved, not cancelled or deleted, because they are important as learning experiences.

Soul fragments, which are essences of powerful soul emotion that have either been left behind, lost or taken on from another person are held on this level. Soul fragments are automatically resolved, cleaned and returned when the practitioner witnesses them so (*see pages 208–209*).

Location
The history level is held in the etheric energy field around the back of the head and shoulders.

THE SOUL LEVEL

Our soul is more divine and expansive than our body. It is like a huge ball of beautiful magnificence that is in one way frail and in another way stronger than one might realize. It is glorious. It is part of God, of the Creator, and is a thing of perfection. The programmes that exist on the soul level are very deep and powerful. They are pulled off the completeness of the individual.

PROCESSES OF THE BELIEF LEVELS

Now we will look at removing and replacing belief programmes on all of the levels.

> Θ *Do not begin the subconscious reprogramming belief work until you have read the remaining chapters in this book. ThetaHealing is a mosaic of different pieces that creates a full design. Each piece builds upon the last. The reading is the basis of the healing, the healing is the basis for the belief work, and the belief work is the basis for the feeling work. Once you have an understanding of each aspect, the concepts will come together.*

THE CORE LEVEL

'Zip Them Up'
The first step is to 'zip the client up', pulling their electromagnetic field together so that they will energy test correctly.

1. Sit down opposite the client. With an up and down motion, move your hand in front of their chest, making a slicing motion downwards and back up again.
2. Energy test them to see if they are hydrated.

Energy Testing
We will start by energy testing, using a choice of three programmes: 'I am beautiful,' 'Healers are evil' and 'I love myself'. The reason that I use these programmes in the beginning is because they are generic programmes that most people share who have not done belief work:

- Most people do not believe that they are beautiful. On a deep level they believe that they are ugly, or that it is wrong to be beautiful.
- The programme of 'Healers are evil' is often a programme of fear due to healers being persecuted.

- The programme of 'I love myself' is one of the things that the healers on this Earth are supposed to learn, achieve and teach others, because no person can completely love another person until they first learn to love themselves.

Energy test as follows:

1. Instruct the client to hold their thumb and finger tightly together. Have them say aloud, 'I love myself.' If their fingers pull apart, this indicates a 'no' response. If they are using Energy Testing Method 2, they are standing up and will lean backward on their heels to indicate a 'no' response.

2. The 'no' response means that the client does not love themselves on one of the belief levels. Energy test to discover which level the programme is on, with the client saying:

'The programme of "I love myself" is on the core level.' (Yes/No.)

'The programme of "I love myself" is on the genetic level.' (Yes/No.)

'The programme of "I love myself" is on the history level.' (Yes/No.)

'The programme of "I love myself" is on the soul level.' (Yes/No.)

If a programme is found on one specific level, it does not indicate that it exists on any other. To find if it does exist on more than one level, you must explore each individual level with energy testing.

If the person you are working with does not energy test negative for one of these programmes, then test one of the other programmes instead.

Releasing and Replacing Programmes

> *Remember that only a positive affirmation is understood by the subconscious. So if you find the programme 'I am afraid', it is not advisable to replace it with 'I am not afraid'. Replace it with 'I am brave'.*

If the person energy tests 'no' for 'I love myself' on all four of the belief levels, this indicates that the belief of 'I love myself, no' exists on all levels. You must ask for verbal permission from the client to release and replace the programme of 'I love myself, no' from the core level and then release and replace it as follows:

TRAIN THE BRAIN: THE PROCESS FOR THE CORE LEVEL

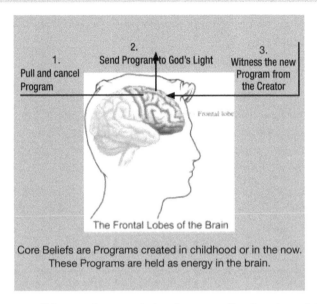

Core Beliefs are Programs created in childhood or in the now.
These Programs are held as energy in the brain.

1. Centre yourself in your heart and visualize yourself going down into Mother Earth, which is a part of All That Is.

2. Visualize bringing up energy through your feet, opening up all of your chakras as you go. Continue going up out of your crown chakra in a beautiful ball of light, out to the universe.

3. Go beyond the universe, past the white lights, past the dark light, past the white light, past the jelly-like substance that is the Laws, into a pearly iridescent white light, into the Seventh Plane of Existence.

4. Make the command: *'Creator of All That Is, I command that on the core level the programme of "I love myself, no" be pulled from [person's name], cancelled and sent to God's light, and replaced with "I love myself". Thank you! It is done. It is done. It is done.'*

5. Imagine going down into the brain to the command centre. This is right at the top of the forehead where the neurons of the brain create programmes just like a computer. Witness the programme and energy associated with 'I do not love myself' being pulled, cancelled and sent to God's light. From the right side of the brain you will witness a magnificent energy burst of negative neurons being pulled and replaced with the new programmes by the Creator. If the change is not witnessed, the programme will not clear and it will rebuild itself into the other levels.

6. As soon as you envision the process as finished, rinse yourself off, put yourself back into your space, ground to the Earth, draw the Earth energy up to your crown and make an energy break.

7. For validation that the programme has been released, energy test with the client saying aloud, 'I love myself.' If their fingers remain pressed tightly together, this indicates a 'yes' response and this means that the programme has been released and replaced on the core level. If they are using Energy Testing Method 2, they are standing up and will lean forward to indicate a 'yes' response.

Congratulations! You have successfully released and replaced your first belief programme!

> Θ *Let me remind you that you must have verbal permission for every individual programme that is released and replaced. Permission to change one programme doesn't give you the right to change another without further permission.*

THE GENETIC LEVEL

Our ancestors have kindly handed down many belief systems on the genetic level. An excellent example of a genetic belief system is the hatred that can sometimes be felt when a white person walks into certain black communities, or when a black person walks into certain white neighbourhoods. These feelings of resentment and hatred have lingered for centuries. Why does one group of people hate another? It makes no sense at all, unless you go back and look into their genetics. The genetic and history levels can both carry beliefs of genetic hatred that can be released with belief work.

For this process to be successful, you must journey into the brain to the pineal gland. It is located directly in through the top of the crown, behind the third eye in the centre of the brain. Inside the pineal is the master cell, the control centre that tells the other cells of the body what to do. Within the master cell is the morphogenetic field, which, you will remember, is the energy field around the DNA of the master cell. You travel into the master cell to witness the process as the programme is released, cancelled, sent to God's light and replaced with the positive belief. This step is crucial for the healing. You will witness the energy of the programme leaving from the right side of the brain (your left side) with a spinning energy. As the programme leaves the body, the energy is sent to God's light. Almost simultaneously it will be replaced with a positive programme, or the correct programme that the Creator brings in. You will see energy swirling downward, flowing into the morphogenetic field of the client from the Creator. When this swirling motion subsides, the healing is done. For the process to be complete, you must witness this whirling motion until it comes to a close.

We will continue with the same client and assume that they stay hydrated for energy testing.

TRAIN THE BRAIN: THE PROCESS FOR THE GENETIC LEVEL

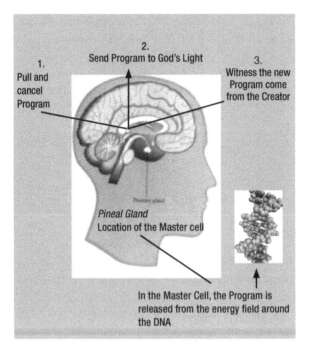

2.
Send Program to God's Light

1.
Pull and cancel Program

3.
Witness the new Program come from the Creator

Pineal Gland
Location of the Master cell

In the Master Cell, the Program is released from the energy field around the DNA

The energy testing has indicated that the programme of 'I love myself, no' exists on the genetic level. Now you will facilitate the belief work to remove the programme of 'I love myself, no' and replace it with 'I love myself' on the genetic level.

Ask for verbal permission to release the programme of 'I love myself, no' and replace it with 'I love myself' on the genetic level.

1.   Centre yourself in your heart and visualize yourself going down into Mother Earth, which is a part of All That Is.

2.   Visualize bringing up energy through your feet, opening up all of your chakras as you go. Continue going up out of your crown chakra in a beautiful ball of light, out to the universe.

3.   Go beyond the universe, past the white lights, past the dark light, past the white light, past the jelly-like substance that is the Laws, into a pearly iridescent white light, into the Seventh Plane of Existence.

4.   Make the command: *'Creator of All That Is, I command that the programme of "I love myself, no" be pulled from [person's name], cancelled and sent to God's light, and replaced with "I love myself". Thank you! It is done. It is done. It is done.'*

5. Imagine going into the brain to the morphogenetic field around the master cell within the pineal gland. Witness the spinning energy burst of the programme being released from the morphogenetic field and sent to God's light and the new programme being replaced by Source.

6. As soon as you envision the process as finished, rinse yourself off, put yourself back into your space, ground to the Earth, draw the Earth energy up to your crown and make an energy break.

7. For validation that the programme has been released, have the client say aloud, 'I love myself on the genetic level.' If their fingers remain pressed tightly together, this indicates a 'yes' response and this means that the programme has been released and replaced on the genetic level. If they are using Energy Testing Method 2, they are standing up and will lean forward to indicate a 'yes' response.

Congratulations! You have successfully released and replaced your first genetic programme! Replacement of the negative belief with the new programme will alter the way that person feels about love instantly.

If you are ever having problems visualizing when you are doing readings or healings, keep your eyes closed and move them slightly upwards towards the top of your forehead, looking upwards towards your crown, and you will see things more clearly.

When you change belief systems in the morphogenetic field, some illnesses and diseases can heal instantly. One of my clients was suffering from cancer of the colon. This was his third bout with this illness. After releasing the belief of 'I hate my father' from his core and genetic levels, he found his cancer disappeared.

THE HISTORY LEVEL

This level is important because the thoughts, memories and information that enter through this doorway need proper discernment and balance. The history level gives us a means of balancing intuitive information that comes to us from undefined origins. Memories are carried in the subconscious mind, in the genes or in the morphogenetic field, but with some memories we have a difficult time identifying exactly where they originate. These are called past-life memories. We call this the history, rather than past-life, level, however, because we are not quite sure if these are deep genetic memories of pure energy, memories of people that we have remote viewed or been in direct contact with, or memories of other times and places such as past lives.

- The history level is pure energy that is a part of the auric field that surrounds the body.
- It is the doorway to all of the lives that we exist on in the past, present and future simultaneously; it's an opening into time and space that we live with every day.
- It is connected to the massive energy of the soul.

Soul Fragments

The history level is a means of returning to reclaim soul fragments. Do not be alarmed about the loss of fragments of your soul. These can be returned to you with a simple command process.

Let me explain. Your soul essence is enormous and connected to the Creator. The soul is here to experience and learn the lessons of the physical body and emotions. In this learning process it extends itself into another person's space and leaves behind a residual essence. The returning and releasing of these essences will strengthen and balance the soul and its instrument, the body, to return all that we are to the All That Is of the soul.

A soul fragment is a shard of essential life-force energy that is lost in emotional encounters. Soul fragments may have been left behind in another place or time. These may be genetic memories that your ancestors lost in a traumatic situation. You may call for any soul fragments that belong in this time to be returned in the highest and best way.

When you are in a romantic situation or any circumstances that will allow you the opportunity to share DNA, you will also leave behind soul fragments. In the long-term care of a loved one that is ill, such as a sick child, it is likely you are leaving soul fragments behind. The soul in its compassion leaves a life force to keep the child alive. In a later chapter there is a soul fragment exercise to release and return specific essences to you (*see pages 208–209*). When the beliefs of the history level are resolved and replaced, soul fragments pertaining to those beliefs are automatically returned.

Past Lives

In the journey of the soul through existence, the essence of other incarnations that are brought into this life is explained by the concept of past lives or reincarnation.

The concept of past lives comes largely from the teachings of Hinduism. Paramahansa Yogananda and other Hindu teachers have stimulated people of the West with spiritual ideologies from India. The spiritual landscape of Western society is one of awakening, and it has been awakening for over 100 years.

The love affair that we have today with the largely Hindu concept of past lives stems from the idea of reincarnation. Reincarnation is a process defined by belief in the immortal soul and the concept of karma. Karma is the teaching tool for the soul. Because certain karma can only be resolved in the physical body, a cycle of reincarnation ensues, leading the soul on a path of learning from life to life.

There are many instances of people having past-life experiences, particularly children. Exactly where the experiences come from is a question open to debate. I am not particularly interested in it, although I will offer some explanations, but past-life memories are very real. I believe that they could come from many different sources.

First of all, we all have DNA memories – memories in the cells that retain the experiences of our life and are passed down from generation to generation. We know that DNA memory goes back at least seven generations. It retains everything that your grandmother and grandfather did before your birth. It is likely that it is accountable for some of what we call past-life memories.

There is a place that we can access called the Hall of Records, or the Akashic Records. These records are said to have existed since the beginning of Creation. They form the library of all events and responses concerning human consciousness in all realities. Every human contributes and has access to the Akashic Records and it is possible to travel to the Hall of Records with your consciousness to view the memories and experiences of each individual. I have personally experienced the Hall of Records, so I assume that others are connecting to it as well. This too is an explanation for many past-life memories.

Also, the land in and of itself holds memories of its own. These memories, or ghost imprints, can be apparent to an intuitive person and can be confused with past lives. (*For further information on ghost imprints, refer to Chapter 20.*)

Last but not least, it is possible that you actually had a past life. It is also possible that you didn't learn everything in that life and it was necessary to live another because of karma. But suppose you did live another life, does it really matter? Reincarnation is not specifically what these Theta teachings are concerned with. We intend to teach something that works with and benefits all religious belief systems.

I believe that we can learn from all experiences, but we are in this life and this is the one that counts. So, be focused on this life. I have had personal experiences with past lives, but I am always careful to keep focused on the life that I am leading now. Don't become caught up in who you were before, what you did or what you experienced. Don't be over-concerned about an existence in another time or place. The most important thing that you must have when you are doing readings or any of these Theta techniques is a belief in the Creator of All That Is. The most important thing to remember is to follow the truth: that *we are all connected to the complete whole.* It is this whole, this completeness, this Creator that we call upon in doing this work. Allow others to believe the way they choose, but don't waste your time trying to analyze things that are of no importance. Use your time wisely living in the present time, in the *now.* Release the past and live in the present. I am not saying you shouldn't remember the past or that you shouldn't learn from the past, but don't get stuck there.

The other reason that I don't agree with the conventional belief in past lives is because my concept of them is completely different. I believe that the souls of those people who have past lives experience past and future lives all at once. This is because I believe that time as we perceive it does not exist. Our past, present and future lives all exist outside our perspective of time. When we are in the right state of mind, however, we can experience some of these overlapping memories.

We will continue with the same client and assume that they stay hydrated for energy testing.

TRAIN THE BRAIN: THE PROCESS FOR THE HISTORY LEVEL

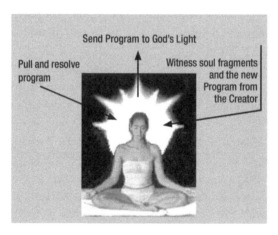

The energy testing has indicated that the programme of 'I love myself, no' exists on the history level. Now you will facilitate the belief work to remove the programme of 'I love myself, no' and replace it with 'I love myself'.

> *NB When changing programmes within the history level it is not advised to make the command using the word or thought form of cancel; always use resolve. This is very important for the process to work correctly.*

Ask for verbal permission to release the programme of 'I love myself, no' and replace it with 'I love myself' on the history level.

1. Centre yourself in your heart and visualize yourself going down into Mother Earth, which is part of All That Is.

2. Visualize bringing up energy through your feet, opening up all of your chakras as you go. Continue going up out of your crown chakra in a beautiful ball of light, out to the universe.

3. Go beyond the universe, past the white lights, past the dark light, past the white light, past the jelly-like substance that is the Laws, into a pearly iridescent white light, into the Seventh Plane of Existence.

4. Make the command: *'Creator of All That Is, it is commanded that the history programme of "I love myself, no" be pulled from [person's name], resolved and sent to God's light, and that all soul fragments be washed and cleaned and replaced with "I love myself". Thank you! It is done. It is done. It is done.'*

5. Witness the energy of the programme of 'I love myself, no' be pulled, resolved and sent to God's light and all soul fragments being washed, cleaned and replaced with the new programme of 'I love myself'.

6. To visualize this level, you must command to be taken to the history level by saying, *'Creator of All That Is, it is commanded to be taken to the history level of [person's name].'* You will be taken to a place that is a little above the person's head and shoulders and you will actually see memories of their past lives, or humankind's history, flash before you. This is the auric field around the body, where the energy is resolved. It is very important when working on this level to remember what issues you are working on. This level is seductive in its beauty. When going into past-life memories, there will be visions and an incredible amount of information. It is easy to be overwhelmed and forget why you are there in the first place. Stay focused upon the issue at hand and make sure it is taken care of before you leave.

7. As soon as you envision the process as finished, rinse yourself off. Put yourself back into your space, ground to the Earth, draw Earth energy up to your crown chakra and make an energy break.

For validation that the programme has been released, have the client say aloud, 'I love myself on the history level.' If their fingers remain pressed tightly together, this indicates a 'yes' response and this means that the programme has been released and replaced on the history level. If the person is using Energy Testing Method 2, they are standing up and will lean forward to indicate a 'yes' response.

Congratulations! You have successfully released and replaced your first history programme!

THE SOUL LEVEL

Over an extended period of time, the Creator of All That Is trained me in the belief work. As I explored the new knowledge, I began to energy test for beliefs that I might have. At this time I had only learned of the first three levels of belief. I found that my body had the programme 'I am crying inside' and this programme would not release from the core, genetic and history levels. The Creator of All That Is told me that it went all the way to the soul level. I was discouraged and upset. I could not understand why it had gone all the way to my soul level. I felt that once it had reached my soul, it was there forever.

The sweet voice of the Creator came into my head and said, 'Vianna, go up and command to release the belief of "Crying inside".'

I replied, 'I can't! It's all the way to the soul level.'

The Creator responded in a calm voice, saying, 'Vianna, your soul is still learning. It is learning and it can be directed towards what it is supposed to experience in this existence for spiritual growth. This is one of the reasons you are here – to learn and experience what you create. Go up and command to release the belief of "Crying inside". You can do no good for yourself or anyone else with this belief. If you are busy feeling sorry for yourself and everyone else, you will have no time left to help anyone. Go up and change it.'

I did as the Creator suggested. I went up above my space to the Creator of All That Is and commanded all soul programmes of 'I am crying inside' to be pulled, cancelled and replaced with 'I have joy'.

I went up to witness the process. When it had finished I experienced a deep, peaceful feeling, down to the very depths of my heart and soul. I felt a change coming over me as it flowed through my body and then expanded outward. I wanted to weep with joy.

There are not many feelings, thoughts and beliefs that are carried to the soul level, but those that do can and will have a profound effect on your life. As you begin to understand the soul level, you will learn how to bring all four levels together in synchronicity to release and replace beliefs instantly. This will enable you to work on each of them in a sequence during a reading or healing.

We will continue with the same client and assume that they stay hydrated for energy testing.

TRAIN THE BRAIN: PROCESS FOR THE SOUL LEVEL

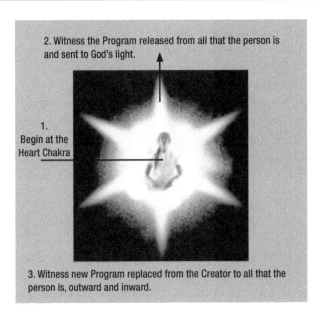

2. Witness the Program released from all that the person is and sent to God's light.

1. Begin at the Heart Chakra

3. Witness new Program replaced from the Creator to all that the person is, outward and inward.

The energy testing has indicated that the programme of 'I love myself, no' exists on the soul level. Now you will facilitate the belief work to remove the programme of 'I love myself, no' and replace it with 'I love myself' on the soul level.

You must ask for verbal permission to release the programme of 'I love myself, no' and replace it with 'I love myself' on the soul level.

1. Centre yourself in your heart and visualize yourself going down into Mother Earth, which is a part of All That Is.

2. Visualize bringing up energy through your feet, opening up all of your chakras as you go. Continue going up out of your crown chakra in a beautiful ball of light, out to the universe.

3. Go beyond the universe, past the white lights, past the dark light, past the white light, past the jelly-like substance that is the Laws, into a pearly iridescent white light, into the Seventh Plane of Existence.

4. Make the command: '*Creator of All That Is, I command that the soul belief of "I love myself, no" be released, cancelled and sent to God's light, and replaced with "I love myself". Thank you! It is done. It is done. It is done.*'

5. To work at this level, go to the heart chakra and witness the programme being released outward from the soul, from all that a person is. Witness the energy of the new programme coming in from Source and replacing the old programme, beginning at the heart chakra and moving outward to the auric field until it is done.

6. As soon as you visualize the process as finished, rinse yourself off. Put yourself back into your space, ground to the Earth, draw Earth energy up to your crown chakra and make an energy break.

For validation that the programme has been released, have the client say aloud, 'I love myself.' If their fingers remain pressed tightly together, this indicates a 'yes' response. If they are using Energy Testing Method 2, they are standing up and will lean forward to indicate a 'yes' response.

Congratulations! You have successfully released and replaced your first soul programme!

EXPERIENCE

When you are even more experienced with belief work it will be a simple matter to ask the Creator if a programme exists on more than one level and how deep it goes. The process will become spontaneous and you will simply know where the programme is and how deep it goes. You will also find that you do not need to use energy testing to validate a belief with a 'yes' or 'no' answer from the client.

As your intuitive senses become attuned to the energy of the client, you will begin to recognize the feeling of different belief systems. You will clearly visualize the belief programmes that are presenting themselves and you will hear yes' and 'no' answers to the belief programmes' statements. *The energy testing is primarily for the benefit of the client.*

SYNTHESIS

The next step will be a leap of faith. In this scenario, the replacement programme will be one that is given by the Creator. The practitioner will simply make the command that the Creator replace the programme.

To release and replace beliefs when a programme is on all four levels, begin by energy testing, remembering that this will only give an accurate answer if the person is hydrated.

Assume that you are going to release and replace a programme that exists on all four belief levels at once. We will use the programme of 'I hate people'.

Have the client say aloud, 'I hate people.' If their fingers remain pressed tightly together, this indicates a 'yes' response. If they are using Energy Testing Method 2, they are standing up and will lean forward to indicate a 'yes' response.

The next step is to find how deep the belief programme goes. Energy test the individual belief levels one at a time to discover which level the programme is on, with the client saying:

'The programme of "I hate people" is on the core level.' (Yes/No.)
'The programme of "I hate people" is on the genetic level.' (Yes/No.)
'The programme of "I hate people" is on the history level.' (Yes/No.)
'The programme of "I hate people" is on the soul level.' (Yes/No.)

In this case energy testing indicates a 'yes' response on every level. So the person believes that the programme of 'I hate people' exists on all the belief levels simultaneously.

Ask for verbal permission to release and replace the programme of 'I hate people' on all the belief levels.

Facilitate the belief work to remove the programme of 'I hate people' and replace it with the programme from the Creator in the belief levels as follows:

THE PROCESS FOR SYNTHESIS

1. Centre yourself in your heart and visualize yourself going down into Mother Earth, which is a part of All That Is.

2. Visualize bringing up energy through your feet, opening up all of your chakras as you go. Continue going up out of your crown chakra in a beautiful ball of light, out to the universe.

3. Go beyond the universe, past the white lights, past the dark light, past the white light, past the jelly-like substance that is the Laws, into a pearly iridescent white light, into the Seventh Plane of Existence.

4. Make the command: *'Creator of All That Is, I command that the programme of "I hate people" be released, cancelled, resolved on the history level, released on the others, sent to God's light and replaced with the correct programme from the Creator. Show me on all the belief levels. Show me. Thank you! It is done. It is done. It is done.'*

5. Say, *'Creator, show me the core level.'* Imagine going to the forefront of the brain. Witness the programme and energy associated with 'I hate people' being pulled, cancelled and sent to God's light. From the right side of the brain you will witness a magnificent energy burst when the negative programme is pulled and replaced with the new programme of 'People can be good' by the Creator.

6. Say, *'Creator, show me the genetic level.'* Imagine yourself going into the brain to the morphogenetic field around the master cell within the pineal gland. Witness the spinning energy burst of the programme of 'I hate people' being released from the morphogenetic field and sent to God's light and replaced with the new programme of 'People can be good' by the Creator.

7. Say, *'Creator, show me the history level.'* You will be taken to a place that is a little above the person's head and shoulders to witness the programme of 'I hate people' being pulled, resolved, sent to God's light, and all soul fragments being washed, cleaned and replaced with the new programme of 'People can be good' by the Creator.

8. Say, *'Creator, show me the soul level.'* Go to the heart chakra and witness the programme of 'I hate people' being released outward from the soul, from all that a person is. Witness the energy of the new programme of 'People can be good' coming in from the Creator, beginning at the heart chakra and moving outward to the auric field until it is done.

9. As soon as you visualize the process as finished, rinse yourself off. Put yourself back into your space, ground to the Earth, draw Earth energy up to your crown chakra and make an energy break.

For validation that the programme has been released, have the client say aloud, 'I hate people on all the belief levels.' If their fingers easily release, this indicates a 'no' response. If they are using Energy Testing Method 2, they are standing up and will lean backward on their heels to indicate a 'no' response.

Congratulations! You have successfully released and replaced a programme from each of the levels!

WORKING ON ALL THE LEVELS SIMULTANEOUSLY

As you begin to understand the belief work, you will be able to work on all four levels at the same time. It will not be necessary to make separate commands for every programme on each level. Eventually the process will occur as fast as thought.

You should first accustom yourself to removing programmes from each individual level so that you train the brain to know where they are. Once the brain is trained and knows the levels, you can remove programmes from all four levels at once as follows:

THE PROCESS FOR ALL THE LEVELS SIMULTANEOUSLY

1. Ask permission to release and replace the chosen programme.

2. Centre yourself in your heart and visualize yourself going down into Mother Earth, which is a part of All That Is.

3. Visualize bringing up energy through your feet, opening up all of your chakras as you go. Continue going up out of your crown chakra in a beautiful ball of light, out to the universe.

4. Go beyond the universe, past the white lights, past the dark light, past the white light, past the jelly-like substance that is the Laws, into a pearly iridescent white light, into the Seventh Plane of Existence.

5. Make the command: *'Creator of All That Is, I command to remove the programmes of [name programmes] from [name person] on all four levels at one time.'* Command that these programmes be pulled, cancelled and replaced on all levels, except on the history level; on this level the programme must be resolved and replaced with what is correct. *'Show me. Thank you! It is done. It is done. It is done.'*

6. Go into the person's space and visualize all four levels presenting themselves at one time.

7. Visualize the programmes of energy being cancelled from all four levels, resolved on the history level and sent to God's light. Visualize the new programmes of energy flowing in from God's light and being placed on all four levels.

8. Stay in the person's space until you are sure the work is finished.

9. Rinse yourself off. Put yourself back into your space, ground to the Earth, draw Earth energy up to your crown chakra and make an energy break.

Even if a belief does not exist on every level, it is permissible to command that belief systems are released from every level at once, but you must always witness them being released and replaced from each and every level, going through the core, genetic, history and soul levels respectively. If you do not witness the change, the belief will not clear.

You may also witness soul fragments being released and replaced on every level. This is a common occurrence in belief work.

I am often asked, 'Can you just command all negative programmes to be changed in your life instantly?' Unfortunately, you cannot. This is because your subconscious does not know the difference between a negative and a positive programme. This is where the conscious mind comes into play to make the decision as to what is negative or positive.

12

THE CREATION OF FEELINGS

When I first began to use belief work in sessions, I was working with a woman who was chronically depressed. She had never been in anything other than in a state of depression. I decided to pull the belief of 'Life is sad' and replace it with 'Life is joyful'. But when I witnessed the process, it was stopped in motion. Her body refused to accept the belief.

When I asked the Creator why, I was told that she had never experienced the feeling of joy and did not know what it was. This piqued my curiosity and I asked the Creator if I had ever experienced joy. I was told no, I had never experienced joy either. This made me frantic! I thought, 'Oh my gosh, I must find my joy. I have lost it somewhere!'

When I had finished the session and had a moment to meditate, I sat down and began to converse with the Creator. The first question that I asked was, 'Creator, would I find my joy if I went to Hawaii?' Of course, the Creator said, 'Yes.' The reason that I asked this question was that I had previously visited the islands and while there had found a degree of peace for the first time. I thought that since I had found peace there, perhaps I could find joy there too.

At the end of my day I went home and told my husband Guy that I needed to take a break and relax so that I could find my joy. My patient husband laughed and said, 'Well, if you have to go find your joy then I'd better not go with you, because you know I have to be moving all the time and you'll be able to relax better without me.' Since someone needed to stay at home and mind the office and store, we agreed that Guy would stay behind and I would go to Hawaii to find my joy.

I had fallen in love with Hawaii and it was to Hana, on Maui, that I was drawn. Against the advice of my husband I decided to go with my friend Chrissie and her three-year-old boy Caspian. Guy knew that Caspian was a bit of a challenge and thought that I would not get any rest with a young child around. I spoke to Chrissie about Caspian and she reassured me that she would watch him closely. Being the optimist that I am and wanting to share Hawaii with my friend, I decided to go with them.

Needless to say, Guy was right about Caspian coming along. On the plane ride to Maui he screamed for 40 minutes non-stop. From the minute we took off from Honolulu until we landed in Hana, he yelled his little lungs out. We landed in a torrential downpour and when we got to our little house, poor Chrissie stressed me out because she worked so hard to keep Caspian out of my way that she was more stressful that he was. Guy had told her I had to relax or else, but neither Chrissie nor I knew how to relax or what it felt like. We drove ourselves absolutely crazy trying to relax.

After three or four days of this, I had not found my joy and it was almost time to go home! The rain finally stopped and the last thing that Chrissie and I did before we left was visit a Heiau-Luakini. This is a sacred Hawaiian spiritual structure that was built centuries ago in honour of the kings and gods. As we walked up to it, I could see that it was a giant pyramid-like structure made of beautiful round stones. I was told that it had been built by all the members of the community in a group effort full of love and joy. Each stone was handed from one person to another from many miles away to the hill of the Heiau. As each stone was placed to build the monument, it was blessed as it was laid to rest.

As I walked alone in the quiet serenity of the ancient monument, I connected to the *feeling* of the place and instantly felt a sensation that I had never experienced before. I realized that this was *joy*. I had never felt it before. I had felt happiness when my children were born, but I had led a poignant life and joy had not been a part of my past experiences.

Then I made the quantum leap: perhaps the Creator could show me how to help others to find joy. I went up out of my space and connected to the Creator and asked how this might be done and I heard a voice that told me, 'Vianna, all you have to do is command to *know*. Ask to know what joy *feels like* and your cells will learn. You are on Earth to learn by experience, but there is no law that says you have to learn through an extended experience. You can learn feelings instantaneously: what joy feels like, what compassion feels like, how to have compassion for yourself, how to have self-love and so on.'

It was at this moment that the feeling work was born. When I got home from Hawaii I had another session with the lady who was depressed and could not feel joy. I taught her what joy felt like from the Creator of All That Is of the Seventh Plane. From that moment on the door was opened to enable people to have feelings they had never had before, such as love, joy, happiness, compassion, forgiveness and respect.

THE FEELING WORK

With the feeling work you can learn not only what a feeling *feels like*, but that it is possible to have it, how to have it and how to use it.

The feeling work is one of the most powerful techniques in ThetaHealing. The speeds at which changes are made with this work are amazing. People can be taught quickly what it *feels like* to be loved, honoured, respected, cherished, even what it *feels like* to live *without* a negative feeling created by habit, for instance 'I know how to live without being miserable'.

As with the belief work, the practitioner energy tests the client, or themselves, to find out if they have or have not experienced specific feelings. Some people have never experienced the certain feelings in their lives. Perhaps they were traumatized as a child and did not develop these feelings, or 'lost' them somewhere in the drama of this existence. This is the reason why when we want to manifest a soul mate in our life, or abundance, or many other things, they do not come about – we have to *experience* what it feels like before we can bring it into our reality.

In order to have feelings such as joy, for instance, or the experience of loving or being loved by someone, or knowing what it *feels like* to be rich, a person must be shown by the Creative Force.

To facilitate this process, get the person's verbal permission, connect with the Creative Force, use the command process and witness the energy of the feeling being 'downloaded' from the Creator and flowing through every cell of their body and on all four belief levels. Once this feeling has been experienced, the person is ready to create life changes.

In this way, what might take lifetimes to learn can be learned in seconds. Do you know what it *feels like* to live without compulsive misery, fear, anger, frustration and conflict? Living with these things can become such a habit that we no longer know how to live without them, even though we cannot truly live with them. The Creator of All That Is can teach you what it feels like to live without these them on every level of your life instantly, and remove fears that have become out of control. This doesn't mean that when you need to feel fear or anger you won't have it, only that you won't have to create fearful situations in your life.

As with the belief work, use energy testing procedures to ascertain what a person does not understand how to feel or what they do not know.

Below is the beginning of a list of 'feelings' and 'knowing' to energy test for (the full list of feelings is in the *DNA 2 Advanced Class Manual*):

'I understand what it *feels like* to have joy.'
'I understand what it *feels like* to be accepted.'

'I understand what it *feels like* to forgive.'
'I understand what it *feels like* to trust my intuition.'
'I understand what it *feels like* to be completely respected.'
'I understand what it *feels like* to forgive myself.'
'I understand what it *feels like* to be on this Earth.'
'I understand what it *feels like* to be connected to this Earth.'
'I understand what it *feels like* to be worthy of God's love.'
'I *know how* to be happy.'
'I *know how* to live without being miserable.'
'I *know how* to live without being angry.'

THE FEELINGS PROCESS

1. Centre yourself. Begin by sending your consciousness down into the centre of Mother Earth, which is a part of All That Is.

2. Bring the energy up through your feet, into your body and up through all the chakras. Go beyond the universe, past the white lights, past the dark light, past the white light, past the jelly-like substance that is the Laws, into a pearly iridescent white light, into the Seventh Plane of Existence.

3. Make the command: *'Creator of All That Is, it is commanded to instil the feeling of [name the feeling] into [person's name] through every cell of their body, on all four belief levels and in every area of their life, in the highest and best way. Thank you! It is done. It is done. It is done.'*

4. Witness the energy of the feeling flow into the person's space and visualize the feeling from the Creator being sent as a waterfall through every cell of the person's body, instilling the feeling on all four belief levels.

5. When you have finished, move your consciousness out of the client's space through the crown chakra and disconnect by rinsing yourself off, entering your body through your crown chakra. Send your consciousness down into Mother Earth, ground yourself, pull the energy up through your body to the top of your crown and then make an energy break.

The following programmes and feelings are in these categories:

'I understand Creator of All That Is' definition of...'
'I understand what it *feels like* to...'
'I know...'
'I know when...'
'I know how...'

'I know how to live my daily life…'
'I know Source's perspective…'
'I know it is possible to…'

Do you have the following programmes? If you do not, connect to the Creator of All That Is and 'download' these feelings into yourself on all four belief levels. (In the *DNA2 Advanced Class Manual* the complete list of downloads is given.) The teaching of these feelings will have a dramatic effect upon the abilities of the intuitive person and create physical well-being.

Programmes regarding the Creator of All That Is
'I *know* the Creator of All That Is.'
'I *know* that "God" and the "Creator of All That Is" are the same.'
'I *know* it's possible to know the Creator of All That Is.'
'I understand what it *feels like* to know the Creator of All That Is.'
'I understand what it *feels like* to be totally connected to the Creator.'
'I *know* that the Creator of All That Is is totally connected to me.'
'I *know how* to be totally connected to the Creator of All That Is.'
'I *know how* to connect to the Creator of All That Is.'
'I understand what it *feels like* to connect to the Creator of All That Is.'
'I understand what it *feels like* to be worthy of the love of the Creator of All That Is.'
'I understand what it *feels like* to know all things are possible with the Creator.'
'I understand what it *feels like* to deserve the love of the Creator of All That Is.'
'I *know* that I deserve the love of the Creator of All That Is.'
'I understand what it *feels like* to allow the Creator to show me what's in the body.'
'I *know how* to allow the Creator of All That Is to show me what's in the body.'
'I understand what it *feels like* to trust that the Creator will tell me exactly what I'm looking at in the body.'
'I *know how* to trust that the Creator will tell me exactly what I'm looking at in the body.'
'I *know* the difference between listening to the Creator of All That Is and myself.'
'I understand what it *feels like* to know the difference between listening to the Creator and to myself.'
'I understand what it *feels like* to show others they are important to the Creator of All That Is.'

'I *know how* to show others they are important to the Creator of All That Is.'

'I understand what it *feels like* to radiate the energy of the Creator of All That Is to the world.'

'I *know how* to radiate the energy of the Creator of All That Is to the world.'

'I *know how* to live my daily life totally connected to the Creator of All That Is.'

'I understand what it *feels like* to allow the Creator of All That Is to do the healing.'

'I *know how* to allow the Creator of All That Is to do the healing.'

'I *know when* to allow the Creator of All That Is to do the healing.'

Programmes regarding the True Self

'I *know* my true self.'

'I understand what it *feels like* to know my true self.'

'I *know* the perspective of my true self through the Creator of All That Is.'

Programmes to See Yourself

'I understand what it *feels like* to see myself the way the Creator sees me.'

'I *know how* to see myself with the definition of the Creator of All That Is.'

'I *know* it's possible to see myself with the definition of the Creator of All That Is.'

Programmes regarding your Life Purpose

'I *know* the perspective of my life's purpose through the Creator of All That Is.'

'I *know* it's possible to know my life's purpose.'

13

KEY CORE BELIEFS

Now that you have learned how to do the belief and feeling work, here are some quick steps to make your facilitation with a client more effective.

DIGGING

One of the ways in which you can be more effective as a practitioner in a one-on-one session is to use something called *digging*. Digging is energy testing for the key belief that is behind many other beliefs. Here, as a practitioner, you have the opportunity to play the investigator. As you energy test a person, the statements you are given will give you clues to their key belief and therefore how to help them.

It is helpful to visualize the belief system as a tower of blocks. The bottom block is the *key belief* that is holding the rest of the beliefs up. It is the root of all the other programmes above it. Always ask the Creator, *'Which key core beliefs are holding this belief system intact?'*

I once worked on a woman who believed she could not heal herself. As the session unfolded, she said, 'I can't heal myself because I don't deserve to heal myself.' I asked her why she didn't deserve to heal herself and she said, 'Because God doesn't want me to heal myself.' I energy tested her to see if she loved God, and sure enough, she loved God. I asked her if she hated God, and she hated God as well. I asked her why she hated God and after a moment of reflection she said, 'God punishes.' I intuitively knew that this was the key to the belief system. Once I had permission, I went into the Theta state and witnessed the belief system of 'God punishes' sent to God's light and replaced with the belief system 'God is a forgiving and loving God'. As the programme of 'God punishes' went to the light of Creation, I witnessed the belief systems of 'I hate God' and 'I cannot heal myself' released as well. All of these belief systems were cleared by releasing the key belief of 'God punishes'.

You will know the key belief has been found when there is a gentle feeling of completion in your heart. You can save hours of time by seeking and clearing the major key beliefs. One of our practitioners suggested visualizing a belief system as a house of cards. You then ask the Creator which key belief system to pull to make the card house fall down, and the belief will become clear to you. As soon as you have the key programme, ask for or find the replacement programmes that are to be installed in the void created by the removed programmes.

It is always best to find the deepest programme of the subject matter you are pulling and replacing before the session is ended.

THE PROCESS TO DETERMINE THE KEY BELIEF

1. Ask the person, 'If there is anything you would change in your life, what would it be?' Then ask them questions about the issue they come up with until you have reached the deepest core issue. You will know that you are close to the key belief when they begin to become verbally defensive, wriggle or cry in a subconscious attempt to hold on to the programme. Pull, cancel, resolve and replace the issue as necessary on whatever belief levels you have found it. The key questions to ask are 'Who?', 'What?', 'Where?' and 'How?'

2. Avoid putting your own programmes or feelings into the investigation process.

3. Be sure you are firmly connected to the perspective of the Creator of the Seventh Plane when you are in the person's 'space'. In some instances, they will loop, hide or take you in circles with the question/answer scenario. Be patient and persistent. It may be necessary to ask the Creator what the deeper programme is.

Energy testing for beliefs involves the functions of both the thalamus and the hypothalamus. The thalamus is located between the brain stem and forebrain. It takes in information such as what is being seen, heard or felt, including touch, pain or temperature. This happens primarily during the waking state. The thalamus compares the incoming information with the stored memories in the cerebral cortex. If no reference is found, the thalamus searches the memory to see what associations or comparisons might be found and makes an intelligent guess.

The hypothalamus keeps the body in balance by controlling the pituitary gland, affecting hormones, metabolism growth and sexual processes. It helps regulate sleep and wakefulness cycles. It influences mood disorders and produces physical changes when the body is threatened as in fight or flight. It also controls the production of sweat, tears and saliva. This is with the eyes open or closed, awake or asleep.

To determine whether you have cleared the key or root programme, test the person with their eyes closed and open. If the belief isn't clear with their eyes open and closed, you have not yet found the key belief, therefore the core belief system of programmes connected to the key belief is still intact. Continue to ask the Creator for the key belief and remove that programme, then retest the client with their eyes open and closed.

REACTION TO BELIEFS

Once you are in the process of seeking a key belief, it must be found before the end of the session or the person may experience a healing crisis. Do not leave them before their belief work is complete, and closely observe them for signs of discomfort. If they feel or act unsettled, or feel any pain or sorrow, then their issues have not been taken care of and the belief work should continue.

If a client experiences inexplicable physical pain in a session it is likely that you are reaching deep subconscious programmes. This means that you are triggering different belief systems that their subconscious is fighting to hold on to. Continue releasing beliefs until the pain has gone. With their permission, ask the person to download what it *feels like* to be safe. Continue with the session until they are comfortable and have a peaceful demeanour.

TEACHING THE MIND BELIEFS

There are two ways to teach the mind beliefs:

1. By pulling and replacing a belief. If you pull a belief you must replace it with a new one.
2. With the feeling work without pulling anything from the client. The person may need more than one feeling.

EXAMPLES OF DIGGING FOR THE KEY BELIEF

Digging for the deepest key belief is easy! All you have to do is ask 'Who?', 'What?', 'Where?', 'Why?' and 'How?' The client's mind will do the digging for you, accessing information like a computer, and will give you an answer to every question. If the client seems to get stuck while finding an answer, it is only temporary. Change the question from 'Why?' to 'How?', etc., until an answer manifests itself. If there is no answer, ask them, 'If you did know an answer, what would it be?' With a little practice, you will learn how to access the ability of the mind to find the answer.

At any time in the belief work process the Creator may come to you and give you the bottom belief that you are looking for, so be open to divine intervention.

Here are some examples of digging.

Digging: Example One
The following is from an actual session:

Man: 'I have a money problem.'

Vianna: '*Why* do you have a money problem?'

Man: 'Because money is the root of all evil.'

(If I were to pull the programme of 'Money is the root of all evil' at this early stage in the reading, it would not affect the deepest or bottom issue.)

Vianna: '*Why* is money the root of all evil?'

Man: 'Because only educated people have money.'

Vianna: '*Why* do only educated people have money?'

Man: 'That is just how it is.'

Vianna: 'If that is true, *who* does that make *you*?

Man: 'I am stupid.'

Vianna: '*Who* told you that?'

Man: 'My father.'

Vianna: '*Why* did your father tell you that?'

Man: 'No, my mother told me that.'

(The brain will find the right memory in order to correct itself.)

Vianna: '*Why* did you think that it came from your father?'

Man: 'I don't know.'

At that point the man began to squirm around uncomfortably in his chair. If a client is looking you straight in the face unflinchingly, without moving their eyes, it is not likely that you are on the trail of the bottom belief. If they become agitated and move around in their chair, on the other hand, you are getting close.

Vianna: 'But *what* if you did know?'

Man: 'They never wanted to have a child; they never wanted a child at all. I am a mistake.'

'I am a mistake' and 'I am wanted, no' are most likely the key or bottom issues here.

To test that the bottom issue has been found, energy test the client with their eyes open as well as with their eyes closed. Then go up and ask the Creator if these beliefs are the bottom issues.

In this case, now release the beliefs of 'I am wanted, no' and 'I am a mistake' and replace them with the belief 'I am wanted'. Be sure to follow up with the feeling work to teach the person what it *feels like* to have the Creator's definition of being wanted. The wording in the command would go something like this: 'I know the definition of the feeling of "I am wanted" from the Creator of All That Is from the Seventh Plane of Existence.' With the client's permission, then instil the feeling from the Creator of All That Is into them.

Once you have found the bottom belief, the digging process will always end up with feeling work to complete the session. This is because if you do not understand what it *feels like* to have a particular programme, simply replacing a programme will only make the mind go in circles.

In this example, at the end of the session bring in what it *feels like* to be wanted, so that the client knows how to be wanted, what it *feels like* to be nurtured and accepted. It is then likely that the issue will clear.

After teaching the client these feelings, energy test him again, and this time the programme of 'Money is the root of all evil' will have gone. People's issues with money are not tied up with money itself. Money is only paper that we put a value to. People have issues with money when they have issues with self-esteem.

Digging: Example Two
This is from an actual session I had with a woman. I found that she had issues with being a healer. She energy tested positive for the programme of 'I'll be killed for being a healer' and negative for 'I can do healing work'.

Woman: 'I'll be killed for being a healer.'

Vianna: '*Why* will you be killed? *Why* can't you do healing work?'

Woman: 'Because they will kill me.'

Vianna: '*Why?*'

Woman: 'Because it is wrong to tell people what I believe.'

Vianna: '*When* did this start?'

Woman: 'It started in another life. No, it was my mother, in this life. Each time that I told my mother what I believed, she used to slap me.'

Vianna: 'So you will be punished for saying what you believe?'

Woman: 'Oh, always.'

Vianna: 'Do you have issues with your mother?'

Woman: 'Of course. She is awful.'

Vianna: '*Why?* Are you punished each time you say what you believe?'

Woman: 'Always. My father used to punish me, too.'

Vianna: '*When* did this start?'

Woman: 'It started when I was four years old.'

Vianna: '*What* happened when you were four years old?'

Woman: 'I remember telling my mother that it wasn't right to treat my dad the way she did. Then she hit me. Every time I stick up for someone that I love, or I say what I believe, I am punished.'

Vianna: 'Would you like to know what it *feels like* to express yourself without being punished?'

Woman: 'Yes, I would!'

'I am punished' is the bottom belief. So pulling the belief of 'If I say what I believe I will be punished' won't clear the bottom issue. First the person needs to know how to live without being punished. So, download for them the feeling of what it feels like to express themselves without being punished. Once I did this with this client, the original programme of 'I'll be killed for being a healer' was cleared.

FEAR WORK

Many years ago I taught a ThetaHealing certification teachers' seminar in Yellowstone, Montana. One of my students came up to me and accused a man in her group of being 'reptilian' and therefore evil. The rumour spread throughout the class that he was a reptilian spy watching the goings-on of the healers. The student was adamant that he must be expelled from the class. When I was confronted with this, I said, 'All beings deserve to learn Theta work. It will be OK. If he really is reptilian, we will just fix him.'

The people in the class were not happy with this explanation because they were locked into the hysteria of their manufactured truth. They were so busy with the imaginary fear that they actually missed the fact that the man was an old soul from the times of Atlantis and a being of light, not of evil at all. It turned out that he had simply rejected my student's advances, which, for some reason, had led her to believe that he was reptilian. If there was a person with 'reptilian energy' in the class, he wasn't it. His feelings, however, were deeply injured by the group's whispers and false accusations.

Fear causes us to stay in our space and blocks our abilities to heal and be healed. It is the only thing that stops us from accessing the Seventh Plane of Existence.

What is your greatest fear? Compulsive fear may cause a block in healings, readings and manifestations. On one hand, you want to manifest something, yet your fears block it. On the other hand, you can create the very thing that is your greatest fear.

When intuitive abilities begin to accelerate, fear is the greatest danger to the person who uses manifestation prayers. If the intuitive person would give as much power to love, light and balance as they do to fear and hatred, there would be little or no self-sabotage. The intuitive person should recognize how much influence thoughts have over their life.

Fear programmes can also be passed on through the genes or through the history levels. Pull, cancel, resolve and replace these energies as needed.

Programmes of fear occupy a great deal of space and when there is an excess of fear, there are problems in the adrenals and lungs.

There is, however, a natural fear response that a person needs to function in times of an emergency. It is important to separate the 'fear programmes' from this natural emergency response. If a person lives in fear, this is a programme, as are phobias. These can be changed with belief work.

CLEARING FEARS

Fear programmes can simply be removed using belief work. When you are dealing with a person who is overwhelmed by a compulsive fear loop in their mind, follow the fear through a scenario by asking what is their greatest fear and the worst thing that could happen to them. Follow the scenario to a conclusion. Using this process to train the mind of a person to work through a fear loop helps them to understand how to overcome the fear by way of finishing the thought form.

Follow the trail of fear through to its end by asking *why* this feeling came about, *how* it happened and *when* it happened. If you reach an impasse with the process and do not know the direction to follow, just sit quietly watching the person and they will come up with a new trail, perhaps involving another time and place.

As fear is released it will move through the body. Suggest that the client gently touch or tap their thymus (the middle of the chest) and it will release the feeling (cellular memory) of their ancestors or their childhood. The thymus is one of the main places where emotional energy is stored in the body.

To have disappointed God is a big fear for people with programmes about God. Along with this often comes the fear that they will not finish their mission for God. Ask the person if they have a programme of 'I have a mission for God' and investigate to see if they have any fears attached to this mission. Test for programmes of 'God hates me', 'God has turned from me' and 'I fear God'. These are all misguided fears about God.

Through doing thousands of readings, I began to see a pattern of fear programmes. This is the process that developed from those sessions that pertained to fear. These are examples from real sessions from ThetaHealing classes.

Fear: Example One

Practitioner: '*What* is your greatest fear?'

Client: 'I fear being poor.'

Practitioner: '*What* will happen if you are poor?'

Client: 'I'll be on the street.'

Practitioner: 'And *what* if you are on the street?'

Client: 'I'll suffer and die.'

Practitioner: 'And *what* if you suffer and die?'

Client: 'I'll become nothing.'

The real fear is 'the fear of becoming nothing'.

Fear: Example Two

I worked on a woman with a phobia about heights. The programme was 'I am terrified of heights'.

In working with a phobia, you must again guide the mind through the fear labyrinth. Ask, 'What is the worst thing that will happen if you are faced with your greatest fear?'

Woman: 'I will fall off the cliff. It is yellow in colour and there are no trees.'

Vianna: '*When* was the last time this happened?'

Woman: 'I don't know.'

Vianna: '*What* happens then?'

Woman: 'The wagon falls on me.'

Vianna: 'Then *what* happens?'

Woman: 'I am stuck at the bottom of this cold cliff.'

> Θ *When they have this much detail they are remembering a real occurrence. It does not matter where the memory comes from. You must walk them through it so you do not leave them in the middle of their greatest fear.*

Vianna: 'Then *what* happens?'

Woman: 'I die of dehydration. It is awful to die of dehydration. The first thing that happens is that you go blind from your eyes drying up.'

> Θ *Death is not the end when it comes to fear.*

Vianna: '*What* is the worst thing that will happen if you die?'

Woman: 'My children won't be able to see me and I will let them down.'

Vianna: '*What* is the worst thing that will happen if you let your children down?'

Woman: 'I will let God down.'

Vianna: '*What* is the worst thing that will happen if you let God down?'

Woman: 'I will be stuck alone in the dark.'

Vianna: 'Then *what* will happen?'

Woman: 'I will be nothing. I will become nothing if I let God down. I am afraid of the nothing.'

'I am afraid of the nothing' is the bottom programme in most of our greatest fears. In fact, it is one of the greatest fears of humankind. The 'fear of the nothing' is the apprehension that there is nothing after death, that there is no God and that all that we will come to is nothing.

Remove the fear of 'I am afraid of the nothing' and replace it with the programme that the Creator of All That Is brings in. Usually this is 'I am always loved by the Creator'.

Now we take the person back to the tall cliff.

Vianna: 'Think about that tall cliff. Does it make you feel queasy?'

Woman: 'That's strange! It doesn't bother me anymore.'

Remarkably, her fear of heights has now gone. The trail to real fear has been followed to the end. The fear was not of heights, it was of letting her children down, letting God down and becoming nothing.

Fear: Example Three

This woman's greatest fear was of deep water.

Vianna: '*What* is the worst thing that could happen if you were in the water?'

Woman: 'I would drown.'

Vianna: '*What* is the worst thing that could happen if you were to drown?'

Woman: 'I would have to come back again.'

Vianna: '*What* would be the worst thing that could happen if you were to come back again?'

Woman: 'It would never stop. I would have let God down and I would have to come back again.'

Vianna: '*What* would be the worst thing that could happen if you were to come back again?'

Woman: 'It would never stop. I would be in an endless torment of coming back again.'

Vianna: 'Then *what* would happen?'

Woman: 'Then I would have to come back again. I would fail in my mission in life.'

Vianna: 'Then *what* would happen?'

Woman: 'I would come back and drown again.'

Vianna: '*What* would be the worst thing that could happen if you were to drown again?'

Woman: 'I would come back over and over again.'

Vianna: '*What* would be the worst thing that could happen if you had to come back over and over again?'

Woman: 'I would never be finished. I would be trapped. I would never be with God again.'

You can guess that the bottom belief here is 'I will never be with God again'. When you release this programme and replace it with 'I am always in the Creator's presence', the fear of water will clear from this particular person.

> Θ *You must realize that every person is different. So there is no single way to work on beliefs. For example, you cannot pull the programme of 'I fear the nothing' from every person that has a fear of heights. Every person is as individual as every grain of sand on a beach.*

THE THREE RS: REJECTION, RESENTMENT, REGRET

I call these programmes 'the three Rs'. Your mind spends an incredible amount of time on these three issues and if you clear programmes associated with them you will open up enough space in your mind to be able to move objects (telekinesis).

Your brain cells, known as neurons, have receptors for emotion. Whether that emotion is depression or happiness, it is like a 'fix' to your cells. Once a receptor is used to an emotion, it has to have it, just like a drug. So, if you are used to being depressed, you will create depression. But, with proper stimuli, your brain makes new connections all the time and when you do the feeling work you stimulate the brain and add new connections. In the feeling work you learn how to live without specific negative habits and so you give the brain the ability to shut down the receptors that are looking for those negative emotional programmes and make new pathways to positive ones. When we do the feeling work it is wonderful to be able to teach a person what it *feels like* to live without depression, without feeling miserable, without the 'poor me' syndrome, and retrain the neuron receptors to accept joy, happiness and responsibility. After the feeling work, if the former negative emotions reappear in the person's life, the person now has conscious awareness and so can shut down those emotions and open themselves up to the positive ones.

REJECTION

Rejection can influence a person for most of their life. It can prohibit success and the finding of true love. The fear of rejection can cause them to fail before they even start something, and to sabotage themselves in everything they do. Clearing the fear of rejection allows a person to live their life.

RESENTMENT

In the pulling of resentment you have to realize that the brain is similar to a computer. If you pull 'I resent my mother', it may clear at first, but seamlessly transform into a grudge against the mother. The next step is to pull the grudge, but then the person may become uncomfortable because the grudge is keeping them safe. The practitioner must teach the client how to live without resenting the mother, and to know that they are safe to do so. This is why we create grudges – we keep ourselves safe from the people that hurt us so that we are not hurt again. You can pull individual resentments with the belief work, but you must go the extra mile and pull the grudges as well.

Here is a key: every person in your life serves you in some way. If there is a person that gives you a difficult time and presents resistance in your life, perhaps resistance is the way you are motivated.

REGRET

Regret can make you very ill. Failed marriages, marriages that are lonely, being lonely, not telling someone you love them, etc. can all keep you from getting better. Regret will affect your whole body, and your lungs in particular.

If you've worked on someone's beliefs and they have not improved, go back to the three Rs. Removing these will clean up the kidneys, the lungs and the liver.

Programmes of the Three Rs

'I am rejected by [person, situation].' Replace this with 'I accept myself' and 'I understand what it *feels like* to live without being rejected'.

'I resent [this person].' Replace this with 'I release resentment' and 'I understand what it *feels like* to live without resentment'.

'I regret [this situation].' Replace this with 'I am free of regret' and 'I understand what it *feels like* to live without regret'.

14

ADVANCED HEALING PROCESSES USING THE BELIEF WORK

Some of us occasionally scream at the heavens or even mutter beneath our breath, 'Why is God doing this to me?' This is a cop-out. God isn't doing anything to you. God didn't decide to make your life miserable. Like a benevolent parent, God lets us decide what our life will be. God has an energy that we may tap into, but unless allowed in, God lets us live our own lives. How many people know that God can change anything in an instant?

Who is this God anyway? A man? A woman?

How many of you believe that when you die you are going to be judged?

How many of you understand what it *feels like* to know that this world is not a reality? That your spirit and your body are occupying this space, but there is no such thing as really being here? Intellectually, how many of you have the deep intimate realization that everything is composed of atoms and energy?

Do you believe that prostate cancer is worse than the mumps?

Do you believe that breast cancer is worse than chicken pox?

Do you believe that diabetes is incurable?

Do you understand what it *feels like* to have an instant healing from God?

This is why we have the belief work. This gives us the ability to answer these questions of the mind, body and spirit so that we may remove and replace belief systems inside our space and connect fully to *All That Is*.

We also need to practise the ThetaHealing technique, because the more you practise, the more you grow. I have people come to me all the time and say, 'I want to do what you can do!' I always tell them, 'OK, but you are going to have to practise.' Still my students persist and say to me, 'No, I want it all now!' And I patiently say, 'No, it doesn't work that way. You still have to practise so that you can grow.'

The best way to grow is to learn how to *feel*. With the feeling work you will learn to bring in from God certain feelings that it would take a lifetime to experience and to experience them *now* for your evolvement.

As your abilities develop you may walk into a room and intuitively 'see' that someone has something wrong with them. It is not your responsibility to walk up to them and tell them so. You have to respect their free will and wait until they ask you to work with them. It is then that they will be ready to heal.

Some people cannot accept an instant healing because they believe that healing should take time – a day, a week, a month – and the healer must respect this. One thing I found about people who healed instantly was that they understood what it felt like to feel healthy, they understood what it felt like to be loved by God and they understood what it felt like to be worthy of God. If a person does not have these feelings they should be instilled with them. But just because they understand what these feelings are like doesn't mean that they believe that they *deserve* them. It may be necessary to do belief and feeling work with them.

A woman contacted me for a healing and I used belief work with her to have God heal her leg of cancer. Later she showed up at one of my classes very angry with me. It seems that the Creator had healed her leg of cancer but neglected to heal her knee of a painful condition unrelated to the cancer. She was very upset about this. Patiently, I went into her space to do belief work to find out why her knee didn't heal. I found that she had the belief 'It is wrong to ask God for too much' and this had blocked the healing. I was curious and I found that I had this programme as well.

As a healer, you must have patience with all kinds of people. Do you have this kind of patience? Do you understand what this kind of patience *feels like*? And remember that just because you know what something *feels like* doesn't mean you know how to *act* on the feeling.

Many of us do not take that next step of accepting healing because we are afraid. What if you could perform instant healing on anyone you touched? Would the little voices inside begin to whisper, 'Who do you think you are? Only Christ can heal like that!' Little debates like this go on in our minds all the time. If we could eliminate them, we could step into our true connection to God. It is as we become unaffected by the negative and positive, cause and effect, good and bad, that we are able to witness God and not be interfered with by programmes.

People raised in the various religious belief systems of the world may not have a clear view of what God is, who God is and what they believe God will do for them. It is a good idea to explore how you view God, the Creator of All That Is.

It is also important to learn how to influence your mind to be in a particular frame with the following programmes: 'I believe in miracles', 'I'm important enough to God', 'I am totally connected to the Creator' and 'I am always connected to God'.

Once you have acceptance and trust of God's love, healing simply happens.

THE NEW PARADIGM: WHAT SERVES THEM?

I have found that some people use an illness to serve them. So, if you find that a person will not accept healing, explore what it is about their condition that serves them. A good example of this would be the attention someone gets during an illness. When you aren't well, people care about you; they send you presents, take the time to call you and stop by to see how you are doing. If you find someone who is served by a disease in this way, find out what beliefs need to be changed so that the disease no longer serves them.

Some individuals make their disease their whole life and therefore will not heal because the loss of the affliction would be too much for them. In some instances the whole meaning of their existence is to do battle with the disease. Perhaps they receive love, attention or sympathy because of it. Or they become so incredibly focused on healing the disease that once the affliction is gone, they feel lost, because the challenge of overcoming the disease was their only reason to live. The healer must give a person like this a new focus, a new reason to live. Otherwise they may simply replace one affliction with another, so as to have a familiar challenge. Most people have a difficult time with change. Unless they can feel comfortable in their new paradigm, they will go back to the old one. So it is important for the practitioner to search for programmes that create a negative result and to release and replace them in order for the person to accept the healing process.

It may also be that the person does not have certain feelings such as 'I understand what it *feels like* to be healed by the Creator'. So, clear any programmes of fear of disease, as fear may interfere with the healing process, and then download the person with feelings they do not have that pertain to living without the disease.

Another suggestion is to train the person to do ThetaHealing. For some people there is no better therapy than helping others to heal.

FREEDOM FROM OBLIGATIONS

When I first began to teach ThetaHealing internationally I asked someone that I had known for many years to come and work for me. He was a good friend of mine and initially he was reluctant to have a friend as a boss but, with some coaxing on my part, he agreed to work for me.

Please understand that I believe that most situations in life are created for a reason. In time I saw why I had intuitively chosen this friend to work for me. You see, I had chosen him for the negative programmes that we shared, not necessarily for the positive programmes. The interaction between the two of us was interesting and for years followed a strange scenario. When I wanted to take chances to create opportunities, he would become incredibly stressed, telling me that I would fail and that it was not possible for me to accomplish my goals. Naturally, my response to him was, 'Want to bet? Watch me go! It will be done, it is so.'

Up until that time, the only way I knew how to get things done was *through conflict*. So I had drawn to me someone who would help me to accomplish my goals, but not in the highest and best way. Eventually I realized that I was keeping him in my life for the wrong reasons. It goes without saying that both of us were miserable in the situation. Finally it was time to let him go so that he could be happy. I had grown out of the constant need to be negatively challenged.

Take a good look at your own life and observe how people are serving you. Find out *why* they are serving you. Is it because you are a victim, or is it that you need conflict to function? If they are serving you in a negative way to create a positive effect, then perhaps it is time to free them of this obligation. But if you do not release the beliefs inside you that are causing the situation, you will replace it with one that is much the same. For example, if you remove someone from your life and they were serving you, then you will just replace them with someone else.

Take a good look at your own life and observe how people are serving you. Ask yourself these questions:

'Is my shyness serving a purpose?'

'Is another person's aggression motivating me?'

'Is there someone in my life that makes me miserable?'

'Is there someone in my life who constantly tells me I can't do something, or is holding me back and not supporting me? Do I have this person in my life to create a challenge to overcome?'

'Is there someone that is keeping me from moving forward? What would happen if I didn't have this person in my life? Would I be able to move forward or would I replace them with another? What are they making me look at?'

If someone is making your life miserable or sad, free them from this obligation.

Also, free yourself from belief obligations such as 'I can't do it', 'It has to be hard', 'It's too easy', 'It can't be that easy' and 'Everything in life has to be hard to be worth anything'. Search yourself for these programmes and replace them as needed. Instil the feelings of 'I know what it *feels like* to accomplish goals without conflict' and 'I know how to exist without conflict'. Pull the programme of 'This person motivates me by conflict'. Replace this programme with 'I free this person from the obligation of creating conflict in my life'.

It may also be necessary to do feeling work connected to this issue.

ADVANCED PROGRAMMES

SELF-COMPASSION

A wonderful friend of mine once told me that she had spent a little time with a famous Lama. She had asked the holy man what he felt was the single most important thing in life. You would have thought it would be 'To have compassion for others', but the holy man replied, 'It is the company that you keep. The most important thing you can do in this life is to keep good company.'

We should all take this wisdom to heart. Look around you, at your friends, your family and your associates. Do they make you feel good about yourself or do you permit them to continually drain you? You may wish to re-evaluate your life.

It is a challenge for some people to have the confidence to keep good company. You must first learn to have compassion for yourself, to know what it is and *feels like*. This can be difficult if there are people in your life that block you from loving yourself or others.

Programmes of Self-compassion
Test yourself for these programmes:

'I understand what it *feels like* to have compassion for myself.'

'I understand *how* to have compassion for myself.'

'I understand *what* compassion is.'

SAFETY

Test yourself also for the *feeling* and *knowing* of being safe if your childhood was turbulent and full of violence and uncertainty. Those who were raised in these situations will not have been able to create this feeling because they will never have experienced it for long periods of time. It is important that it is instilled in a person since without it they will unconsciously create situations that are unsafe in thought, deed and action.

Programmes of Safety
'I understand what it *feels like* to be safe.'

'I understand what it *feels like* to feel safe in my human body.'

ACCEPTANCE

Perception of information is an important factor in the understanding of healing. Many factors come into play: background, present state of mind, emotional balance and physical state as well as spiritual development. All these are factors in the ability to listen and discern sacred knowledge.

Learn to fine-tune your perceptions so that you may find the essence of acceptance without the interference of negative and even positive influences that can block development.

Test for 'I accept myself'. This may completely clear you of self-doubt. If you test positive for the programme of 'I have self doubt', change it to the programme of 'I have pure acceptance of self'.

Programmes of Acceptance
'I understand what it *feels like* to be accepted.'

'The Creator accepts me.'

'I understand *how* to accept instant healing from God.'

'I accept my human body.'

JOY

Many of the people that you will work with will not understand what joy *feels like*.

Programmes of Joy
'I understand what it *feels like* to have joy.'

'I understand what it *feels like* to learn from joy.'

LIVING IN THE NOW!

Most people have spent so much time living in the drama of their story that they have forgotten to be in, and live in, the now. These people are often living more in the past than in the present. You may have a wonderful day but not be aware of it until afterwards. Teach yourself to live in the now.

Programmes of Living in the Now

'I am living in the now in this moment and this second.'

'I understand what it *feels like* to live in the now with joy going through my body.'

SACRIFICE

Some people act out commitments from genetics, from history or other planes in other times to re-create major sacrifices in this present time. This is because the soul is growing in the only way it knows how. It needs to be retrained so that it may advance without having to sacrifice everything in order to grow spiritually or to gain materially.

Sacrifice is different from commitment and conviction. Ask God that you may know the difference between these aspects. Sacrifice is a choice. Lastly, we should remember that service is also different from sacrifice.

Programmes of Sacrifice

'It's my job to save the world.' Replace with: 'I am in perfect harmony and balance.'

'I am responsible for everything the world does.'

'I have to sacrifice myself for Jesus to love me.'

'I have to sacrifice myself for anyone to love me.' Replace with: 'I am loved always.'

'I must sacrifice to make money.'

DIVERSE BELIEF SYSTEMS

MONEY

The belief systems surrounding the concept of money are a good way to illustrate how to release and replace negative belief programmes.

For centuries it was believed that people had to be humble to communicate with God. Since those who had money were not looked upon as humble, money was therefore thought to be 'the root of all evil'. Now we realize that the Creator is abundant in all ways.

So let's imagine that you're going to work on someone for programmes relating to money. You've made certain that they are hydrated and ready to test. The first thing you do is energy test them by having them declare whether they believe themselves to be wealthy or poor. Let's say they test positive for 'I am poor'.

After you have received permission from the client, go up to the Creator, make the command, go into their space and witness the belief of 'I am poor' being released and replaced with 'I am wealthy'. Then muscle test again and have them say, 'I am poor.' This time their hands open freely, which is a 'no' answer.

Then begin to energy test for the genetic level. The person again says, 'I am poor.' Once again they confirm, 'Yes, I am poor.' You then know that this belief system is definitely on the genetic level. After you have received permission, the belief system of 'I am poor' is released and replaced with 'I am wealthy' for the genetic level.

As you replace the programme with 'I am wealthy', you may feel a terrible conflict emanating from the client. You quickly test them for the programme of 'Having money is bad'. They respond with 'Yes.' When you test them again they make the statement: 'I took an oath of poverty.' Sure enough, they do have an oath of poverty because they tested positive for 'Having money is bad'. Once permission has been given, go to the history level and command all oaths of poverty to be pulled, resolved and sent to God's light, and all soul fragments be washed, cleaned and replaced with the new programme of 'All oaths are finished now'.

Oaths of poverty are usually made on the genetic level and the history level. It may be necessary to check with the person on a core belief level too, if they have ever been a priest or anything pertaining to that profession in this life.

Energy test the person and see if they still have an oath of poverty on the history level. If not, the next step is to energy test for the soul level. In most instances, issues are not carried to the soul level; however, any programme that is deeper than one level can go as far as the soul level.

I used the subject of money because healers the world over think they should be humble and therefore poor. There is no wisdom, written or otherwise, that says that being humble means living in poverty. Many humanitarian deeds can be accomplished with money. Starving children can be fed and people that are suffering throughout the world can be taken care of. If someone's belief is that money is evil and therefore *having* money is evil, this obviously needs to be released.

STRUGGLE

Another example of a flawed belief system is 'I have to struggle'. I once believed that I had to have struggle in my life. As a consequence I created the first 30 years of my life to be a complete struggle.

This is a programme that needs to be pulled and replaced with 'Life is an adventure'. Interestingly, this programme is carried not only genetically, but occasionally you find it on the history level. Release and replace the programme of 'I have to struggle to receive the good things of life'. It is true that we can learn through all our experiences, but we can learn through good experiences just as easily as we can through bad experiences.

It is quite interesting to observe all the lessons that a healer or spiritual person will put themselves through. In so many ways I am very grateful for the lessons that I have created for myself, as these have enabled me to have empathy for people in all walks of life. However, programmes of struggle can be changed to 'Life has challenges' and 'Life is an adventure'. Do not replace programmes of struggle with 'Life is easy' or the soul gets bored and stops the learning process.

SUFFERING

The concept that we have to suffer to learn is false. We need to embrace the truth that we can experience happiness, challenge and adventure. Life is meant to be an adventure. The soul does not particularly care whether you're having a good adventure or a bad adventure, as long as you are learning. Why not make the journey a joyful experience?

Of course there are certain things in life that you are unable to completely control. The fact remains that you cannot control another person's life, but you can control your own decisions and what you create. Releasing the need to suffer will save you a great deal of time and energy.

Programmes of Suffering
'The more I suffer, the faster I learn.'
'The more I suffer, the closer I am to God.'

'I AM ALONE'

I have found in belief work that people like to hold on to beliefs they perceive as comfortable. I watched one client struggling very diligently to hold on to the belief that she was alone. She made statements such as 'We are all born alone', 'We will all die alone' and 'We are islands unto ourselves.' I explained to her that, in truth, we are constantly surrounded by unseen guardians. We are surrounded by assigned companions and the loving energy of the Creator. We truly are never alone.

When replacing someone's programme, always ask the Creator what to replace it with if you are unsure. You will always get an answer from the Creator. You are never alone in the belief work.

'I AM A VICTIM'

Another belief system that some people hold on to is that of being a victim. Looking back over the people who have attended my classes, I would estimate that easily eight out of ten women have been molested, and probably five out of ten men. This is not something new; this is unfortunate, but real. I include myself in that group of eight out of ten women. But you cannot let it destroy your life or give you the excuse not to live.

Releasing the programme of 'I am a victim' from people is vital for their health and well-being. Energy test the client (or yourself) for programmes of 'I am a victim', 'I am abused' and 'I am molested'. Replacing the belief of 'I am a victim' with the positive affirmation of 'I am a power in my life' or the programme that the Creator tells you to replace it with will change their (or your) life dramatically and permanently!

Teach the person the programme 'I know what it *feels like* to live life without being a victim'.

BEING OVERWEIGHT

It is enjoyable to help people release programmes of being overweight. People are overweight for many different reasons. One reason is that they may feel that they should be overweight because everyone else in their family is obese. Another reason is that they feel that if they are overweight they are safe and protected. Or they may have what is called the 'overweight gene', an interesting belief system in and of itself.

Energy test the person to see if they believe that being overweight is powerful, safe and secure. However, everyone is different and the person may have other beliefs. Hidden beliefs might be 'I am powerful when I am overweight', 'I must gain weight to be intuitive' and 'I am heavy'. Be sure to test for these programmes in the history level. Also be sure to release the programme of 'I am a victim' from them.

In many cultures in the past, being heavy was a sign of wealth, power and prosperity. In some tribes, especially Hawaiian and some Native American tribes, the heaviest person was the most powerful. Energy test the client and see if they have one of these beliefs about being overweight.

Any programme that has to do with 'I am overweight' or 'I am fat' should be replaced with 'I am thin' or 'I am healthy'. You will find that beliefs about being overweight are usually carried at least to the genetic level.

You may have to 'dig' for the bottom belief. Do not be surprised if this belief has nothing at all to do with being overweight.

DUAL BELIEFS

The spiritual subconscious can be a little tricky. I discovered that there are many people who have dual belief systems. A dual belief is two belief programmes that are opposite from one another in their meaning but have the same theme and that exist simultaneously on one or more of the belief levels. For example, when a practitioner is energy testing for belief programmes, the client might test positive for the programme of 'I am abundant' but also test positive for the programme of 'I am poor'. So they believe that they are or can be abundant but at the same time believe they are poor.

To release a dual belief, simply leave the positive programme in place and release the negative programme to God's light and then replace it with the correct positive one.

Bearing in mind the prevalence of dual belief systems, as you energy test for belief programmes you should also test for opposing programmes. For instance, if you energy test for the belief of 'I hate my mother' and the client tests positive for the programme, it is quite possible that they might have the opposing programme of 'I love my mother'. Some people are shocked by the knowledge that they carry hate for their mother as a belief. It is a useful therapeutic tool to show them that they still love their mother and are carrying dual beliefs of both love and hate for her.

Similarly, if a person tests positive for the programme 'I am overweight', test to see if they believe they have the programme 'I am thin'. Or, if they believe they are wealthy, don't continue until you have tested to see if they believe they are poor as well. I found that I believed I was rich and poor at the same time.

Always verify dual beliefs on all the levels.

HATRED AND FORGIVENESS

The word, feeling and programme of hate are one of the most prevalent challenges we have. I believe that hatred is the most prevalent cause of disease. So much energy is given out in hatred that it becomes unconscious. When people harbour hatred and hold it inside it can build up in the body to cause physical disease. Therefore it is essential to release all hatreds from all levels of a person's being, whether of the present or of the past in origin.

Releasing hatred for another person has an immediate effect on the physical body. When you release anything from the morphogenetic or subconscious level you will see a physical change take place in the person. Liberating someone from the belief systems of hatred will improve their health immediately.

I was working with an individual who was very weak. I found the source of his weakness to be his liver. After energy testing him, I decided that the problem was stemming from a hatred of his mother. This hatred was so strong it was affecting the function of his liver. Once I had permission, I went up and commanded that all hatred for his mother be pulled, cancelled and replaced with 'I forgive my mother'. When I had done this, not only did his liver begin to function normally but he was once again able to have a normal relationship with his mother.

Some people, however, cannot be reprogrammed to forgive a certain person. If you encounter someone who will not receive the replacement programme, it means that they are not ready to forgive. If a person does not wish to forgive someone, perhaps someone who molested them, replace the programme with 'I release this person to God's light now'. Don't always force the issue of forgiveness; releasing is forgiveness in its own way. Some individuals must release their feelings before they can forgive someone, or they may need to be taught the feeling of forgiveness.

You should be careful with instilling forgiveness to replace a programme such as 'I hate my father or 'I hate my mother'. In some instances a person is holding on to these programmes to keep these people at bay. Hating and not forgiving them is the only way they have to control their feelings towards them. Perhaps here it is best to release the hate and instil that the person has proper discernment in their feelings toward their father or mother. Be sure that the person understands what forgiveness *feels like* with proper discernment.

As I worked with more and more people, I began to see that many people had deep programmes of hatred. Consequently, I went up and started working on myself. On a conscious level I didn't believe that I could possibly hate anyone ever. But sure enough, my subconscious was hanging on to the past. There were a few people that I didn't like. Once I had released this dislike from myself, I began to feel an inexplicable strength coming back into my body. It was once explained to me that hatred consumes the life-energy of a person. I was told that when you release hatred from your body, you should replace it with a different emotion.

I extended this internal search and tested myself for different people that I knew for programmes of hatred. I discovered that I held hateful feelings towards many people. This was something of a surprise, because I had been brought up to believe that it was wrong to hate and I hadn't thought that I hated anybody. I began to pull these emotions off and replace them.

I challenge you to be honest with yourself. Energy test yourself for subconscious hatred towards anyone who has hurt you. Energy test yourself for hatred of family, old enemies and workmates. You will be surprised at how many people you hate. Be aware that these programmes may be genetic in origin, passed down from generation to generation.

Release the hate, cancel it and send it to God's light to be replaced with 'I release' or 'I forgive':

'I understand what it *feels like* to forgive someone.'

'I *am* good enough to be forgiven.'

'I *know* what it *feels like* to forgive myself.'

Command to know what the feeling of forgiveness *feels like*.

Once you release the hatred, make sure you also set free programmes such as 'I am angry with [person's name]'.

Test also for hidden programmes of self-hate, the programmes 'I hate my family' and 'I hate God', and cancel and replace them as needed.

RELEASING PREJUDICE AND HATRED

Energy test yourself also for unreasonable prejudice towards people.

First of all, energy test for the programme of 'I understand what prejudice means'. If you don't test positive, use the wording '[Someone] offends me'. For example, 'Homeless people offend me'.

Then energy test for the hidden hatreds of prejudices towards other ethnic cultures and peoples, for example: 'I hate white people', 'I hate blacks', 'I hate the Japanese', 'I hate Jews', 'I hate Muslims'.

Energy test for: 'I am prejudiced against or offended by...'

Australians	Chinese	Cubans
Egyptians	Israelis	Italians
Japanese	Jamaicans	Mexicans
Poles	Puerto Ricans	Russians
Saudi Arabians	Spaniards	Taiwanese
Vietnamese	Canadians	Greeks
Irish	Scots	Czechs
Yugoslavians	Romans	Austrians
Mongolians	Indonesians	Polynesians
Danes	The Swiss	Icelanders
Native Americans	African Americans	Caucasians
Germans	French	Afghans
Hispanics	Asians	Americans

British	Indians	Argentineans
Addicts	Alcoholics	Transvestites
Bisexuals	Homosexuals	'Holy Rollers'
Men	Fat people	Doctors
Slender people	The homeless	Psychics
Poor people	Rich people	Prostitutes
Children	Educated people	Elderly people
Sick people	Myself	Women
Pentecostals	Jewish people	Jehovah's Witnesses
Catholics	Born Again Christians	Mormons
Baptists	Protestants	Atheists
Hindus	Muslims	Buddhists

If it is found that the test is positive for these hatreds, pull, resolve, cancel and replace as appropriate. It may not be best to replace the programme with 'I love'. Sometimes it is better to replace it with 'I have proper discernment for' or 'I can love my fellow man'. Understand that you may have no idea that you have these subconscious programmes.

It is not uncommon to be prejudiced against your own ethnic group or religion.

MULTIPLE PERSONALITY DISORDER

When working with a client who has MPD, do not presume to eliminate the personalities you choose to believe are not helpful! Rather, find harmony and agreement amongst the various aspects or personalities of the client. Help the various personalities work together in a positive integrative manner.

When starting belief work with a subject with multiple personality disorder it is important to understand that you may initially be contacting only one of the personas at one time, or pulling the programme for only that single persona. To be effective, the programme must be pulled and replaced for each of the personas. If this is not done, the old programme will be likely to be reproduced by those personas not initially addressed. Therefore, you must ask for verbal permission from all the personas at once before pulling and replacing the programme. You must also persuade any resistant persona to accept the release of the programme.

Go up and connect with the Creator, then go down into the person's space and envision speaking to all the personas to get them to agree to have the particular programme pulled. (Note: Some of the programmes will not be held by all the personas.)

Here is the process:

THE PROCESS FOR MPD

1. Ask permission from all the person's personalities to pull the chosen programme.

2. Centre yourself in your heart and visualize yourself going down into Mother Earth, which is a part of All That Is.

3. Visualize bringing up energy through your feet, opening up all your chakras as you go. Continue going up out of your crown chakra in a beautiful ball of light, out to the universe.

4. Go beyond the universe, past the white lights, past the dark light, past the white light, past the jelly-like substance that is the Laws, into a pearly iridescent white light, into the Seventh Plane of Existence.

5. Make the command: *'Creator of All That Is, it is commanded to resolve on the history level, cancel on the others and send to God's light the programme of [name the programme] and replace it with [name the new programme] from [name the individual personalities] on all four belief levels at once. Thank you! It is done. It is done. It is done.'*

6. Go into the person's space and visualize all four levels coming up at once in all the different personalities.

7. Visualize the programmes of energy being released, cancelled from the core, genetic and soul levels, resolved on the history level and sent to God's light. See the new programmes of energy flowing in from God's light and being resolved and replaced on all four levels of each separate personality.

8. Stay in the person's space until you are sure the work has finished. Rinse yourself off with God's light and put yourself back in your space. Go into the Earth, pull up Earth energy through all your chakras to your crown chakra and make an energy break.

FREE-FLOATING MEMORIES

Free-floating memories are programmes that a person has accepted when the conscious mind has shut down and the unconscious mind has been vulnerable to them. When the words, noise or situation are repeated that were accepted by the person in the unconscious state, they will replay the trauma in the waking world. This generally happens when the person has had a loss of consciousness, as with surgery, accidents, wartime trauma, extreme abuse or excessive alcohol or drug use. If you have a client that seems resistant to healing, check for free-floating memories.

The person with a free-floating memory may have different reactions when the brain is reminded of the programme by a spoken word, a noise or a situation from the point of trauma, ranging from a simple headache to full-blown seizures.

THE PROCESS FOR RELEASING FREE-FLOATING MEMORIES

1. Centre yourself in your heart and visualize going down into Mother Earth, which is a part of All That Is.

2. Visualize bringing up energy through your feet, opening each chakra to the crown chakra. In a beautiful ball of light, go out to the universe.

3. Go beyond the universe, past the white lights, past the dark light, past the white light, past the jelly-like substance that is the Laws, into a pearly iridescent white light, into the Seventh Plane of Existence.

4. Make the command: *'Creator of All That Is, it is commanded that any free-floating memory that is no longer needed, that no longer serves this person, be pulled, cancelled and sent to God's light, in the highest and best way, and be replaced with the Creator's love. Thank you! It is done. It is done. It is done.'*

5. Move your consciousness over to the client and witness the healing taking place. Watch as the old memories are sent to God's light and the new energy from the Creator of All That Is replaces the old.

6. As soon as the process is finished, rinse yourself off and put yourself back into your space. Go into the Earth, pull Earth energy up through all your chakras to your crown chakra and make an energy break.

THE NEW LIFE EXPERIMENT

The New Life Experiment is training ourselves to self-monitor what we say, what we do, how we act and how we react to others. This exercise will show you just how much negativity we create in our lives and how we can stop ourselves from saying and doing negative things.

When you catch yourself using a negative statement, always cancel it. Better yet, catch yourself *before* you say it and choose a different thought. Shift to a different reality and choose to use your energy on your manifesting or healing work.

Negative thought forms consume an incredible amount of energy. So, as a negative thought form begins to take shape, stop it in motion and back up and teach yourself the Creator's perspective on the situation. Send yourself the love and energy to change it with ease and grace to a positive situation. Permit the Creator to teach you how to move forward to take the next spiritual step.

Things to remember:

No complaining.

No whining.

No being overly critical.

No being overly judgemental.

No poking fun at others.

No being cynical or facetious.

No creating reasons to be sorry or to say you're sorry out of habit.

No creating reasons to be stressed.

No creating reasons to be unhappy.

No affirming negative thoughts such as 'I'm overweight.'

No affirming negative feelings such as 'I'm depressed.'

No making reasons to be angry.

No making or seeking out reasons to overcome others, fight, struggle or enter into combat (more than necessary).

No making reasons to be anxious.

No making reasons to be overwhelmed.

No making reasons to worry.

No making reasons for self-doubt.

No creating situations of lack or scarcity with statements such as 'I don't have enough energy.' Instead make the claim 'I have plenty.'

No creating chaos or drama for entertainment, excitement, adventure or thrills, or to avoid peace.

No 'wrong' or 'right', 'better' or 'worse', 'should', 'hope' or 'try'.

15

THE LAW OF TRUTH

I have always been close to the spirit world. From the age of four, I have had spiritual experiences. These experiences have come in a broad range, from apparitions to waking visions. In the early years, they were not necessarily wanted. They would just come out of the blue into my world, appearing with an abruptness that was at times startling.

As I grew older, I began to have more control over these experiences. This was because of my belief in God. I have always felt a deep connection to God. I loved God so deeply that when it came to spiritual experiences, I had no fear of them because I knew that I would be protected. God is over all.

Because of this belief, there was no reason for me to have any fear, doubt or disbelief of things that were spiritual. My intuitive abilities developed unhindered, until I could actually reach out and swirl moon-dust by putting myself in a Theta state.

You see, when you begin to experience a purposeful Theta state, you are in a waking dream state. A dream state enables you to be more receptive to the metaphysical and spiritual world around you. For instance, there are some disembodied spirits that are good, and some that aren't. In the following chapters I'm going to teach you how to tell the difference and what to do with them so that you have no fear. Compulsive fear is just a waste of time. Irrational fear accomplishes nothing. And the only things that stop intuitive healing from working are fear, doubt or disbelief.

In my classes I teach people through stories. This is a little story about when I first met the Law of Truth. It all started with a free reading…

Years ago, before I worked doing readings and massage, while I was still in security, a psychic I met decided to give me a free reading. I have always been intuitive, so I gave her a reading in return. I 'read' the psychic impression on her ring and then took her hand and 'read' her. Apparently, she liked it. She said, 'Honey, you're pretty good at this. You should do this.'

She wanted to leave town to be with her husband, but she was in a lease contract with a massage therapist. She was paying half the rent of their office and the massage therapist told her that if she wanted to leave, she had to find someone to take her place. She asked me if I wanted the office. At that time I had trained in massage therapy and as a naturopath, but I was a little uneasy about leaving my job as a security guard. But I saw it as an opportunity, so I told her that I would take over the lease. I am glad that she saw my potential. It just so happens that she was also the mother of the woman who was to become my best friend, Chrissie.

Two months after I had done the reading on her, I was in my shop offering massage, readings and nutritional counselling. Of the three, it was the readings that took off first, although I gave a good therapeutic massage. In time, I was to fuse the nutritional counselling with the readings. I had to have a couple of appointments a day to make ends meet. Unfortunately, I was soon left with the whole office due to my lease partner becoming pregnant, and I had to come up with not only my half of the lease but hers as well.

I realized that the only way to be a good reader was to be able to see the truth. I knew that I could tell people what they wanted to hear, but if I told them the truth then they would come back, and they would tell other people about me. I felt that this was the only way I could make this work. I remember sending out the prayer, 'God, please, teach me how to see the truth.'

It was a few weeks after this that my answer came. My children were in Utah visiting their father, and my husband at the time was away for police training. So when I came home from work, I was completely alone. I got into bed, went to sleep and found myself in a strange dream. Giant faces were floating in my living room. They were huge! They said, 'Vianna, come with us. We have something to show you.'

Well, of course, I fought my way out of sleep and woke up. I thought, 'That was a weird dream. That was strange.'

Then I got up to go to the bathroom and I saw them in reality – big, huge faces floating in my living room. They were constantly shifting in form; strange energy was flowing from them. Sometimes they looked like huge balls of energy, sometimes faces. For some reason, I could tell that all of them were shifting energy. As one, they said, 'Vianna, come with us. We have something to show you.'

So, of course, I did what any self-respecting intuitive would do: I ran to my bed, crawled under the covers and prayed *really* hard that they would go away!

I continued to pray until finally they did go away. Needless to say, I didn't sleep much for the rest of the night.

This experience was something that I was *not* prepared for.

Up to this point I had read about the human body, anatomy, parasites, vitamins, minerals, God, scriptures and religions, but not very much about metaphysics. Although I had seen spirits before, this was different. The paranormal was part of my life, but this experience was a bit out of my league.

By this time I had developed a friendship with Chrissie. She would come into the shop to talk about all kinds of things. I knew that she had been raised a psychic all of her life and because of this had read all different kinds of metaphysical philosophies and books. I resolved to ask her about the encounter the next day.

The next day, when she came to visit me in the shop, I said, 'You will never believe what happened! I had these really huge faces in my living room and I ran under the covers and prayed and prayed that they'd go away.'

She was excited and said, 'Oh, Vianna, that is so cool!'

Perplexed by her reaction, I said, 'It is?'

Chrissie said, 'Yes, it is! It's wonderful! Vianna, the next time that they visit you you've got to go with them! You've got to find out what they want!'

Puzzled and a little uneasy, I said, 'OK.' I felt confident that I'd prayed hard enough to prevent them from coming back.

Chrissie must have noticed my reluctance because throughout the day she made a point of coming back into the shop on her breaks. She began to tell me about all things metaphysical. She told me about alien visitations, group consciousness and other things. She persisted with this talk throughout the day to hammer her point home. Finally, I promised her that if the faces ever came back again, I would go and see what they wanted. I'm a person of my word.

When I went home that night I searched through my house, just to make sure there was nothing there. I wasn't really expecting to find anything, and I felt pretty confident that the experience would never happen again. I got into bed and curled up to sleep. But before I could get to sleep they came back. They were taller than I was and four of them blended together, first one countenance, then another. They spoke to me and said, 'Vianna, come with us.'

The thought that came into my mind was that I was bound by the promise I had made to Chrissie. Mustering my courage, I thought, 'What is the worst thing that could happen to me? I could die?' I said to myself, 'Alright, fine. We all have to die sometime. What do I have to lose? They're never going to leave me alone; I might as well go and see what they want.'

It was then that I was taken to a place where I saw what looked like rows and rows of hay bales. These bales were hanging down from hooks. The entities told me to touch one of them. When I did, I could see the deepest, darkest secret of everyone that I was working with in my shop. Suddenly, I could see the deepest, darkest secret of *every person in my life*. It was horrible! I saw a woman who had come to me in the shop and who I had felt had some sexual issues. She was molesting her two little children, aged two and four. As I moved from bale to bale, touching each one, I was privy to every evil secret that these people wanted to hide from the world. The vision included everyone I talked to, all my neighbours, every client I had. It was one of the most awful experiences of my life. In fact, it's the reason why I left my second husband. I was in this vision for most of the night and when I had seen my husband's deepest, darkest secret, I was finally released from it.

I was terrified and upset. I had watched a man who was taking care of invalid children molest them on a gurney. I had watched people lie. I had watched people do things that were just unbelievable. The next day, I got up and decided that I was packing up my children and my car and driving to Montana. I would find a little town to live in and talk to people as little as possible. I felt that the whole human race was awful.

Then I realized that I didn't have enough money to set myself up in Montana. I had to go to work to earn the money. My plan that morning was simple: I would get my kids from Utah and once I had enough money I would drive to Montana.

I arrived at work tired and disillusioned. Chris met me there and I told her my experience. She was animated and began to ask me questions. When I told her her deepest, darkest secrets, she validated them.

Even with this validation, however, I let feelings of doubt creep in. What if I had only dreamed it? What if I was only right about Chris? What if I was wrong about the others? What if those things hadn't really happened? What if I had made it all up?

I decided that I needed a second validation. God must have been with me that day, because I received it. In fact God sent me seven people who had been in my vision.

The woman who had molested her little children was the first to come into the shop. The words just fell out of my mouth. I said, 'You molested your own children.'

She collapsed at my feet and started to cry and begged me to forgive her. It was terrible to see. I was mortified because now I had validated what I'd seen, and it was the same awful truth with each client that came in that day.

By the time I had finished with my clients, it was dark and I didn't have time to drive the four hours to Utah, pick up my kids and then turn around to drive the six hours to Montana. So I went home and went to bed.

Just as before, the huge faces came again. Only this time, they had more surprises. I was taken up through what I later came to know as the planes of existence. I rose through the six planes until I reached the Law of Truth. From this lofty place of purity, I could see all the levels of existence that were my life and the lives of all the people in the world. From this place I was shown the deepest, darkest secrets of my life. They showed me everything that I had done in my life.

They also did something to me that at the time I did not fully understand: when they took me up and showed me my life I realized that *I* had made every decision that had led me to where I was now and that *I* was responsible for what was going on in my life. You see, I had grown up in a good Christian home. My view had been that God had given me tests to prove my strength and ability to learn. Because I believed that I could get closer to God through suffering, I had created truly bizarre experiences. The faces showed me that *I* had created them.

At that moment in my life I was with a person that I wasn't in love with, in a place where I didn't want to live and was faced with having to leave my shop because I couldn't meet my financial obligations. I could see all of this and the realization came to me: I had created it.

Then the Law of Truth said, 'Look! You can change anything! All you have to do is *go up and be in this place*. Now look down at yourself, Vianna, down at the energy of your life, and command change and it will be done.'

I said to the Law, 'That's impossible. This can't be true. How can this be true? I spent an entire life creating this mess – do you think I can fix it in 30 seconds or less? That's ridiculous.'

After a brief pause I thought about it and said to the Law, 'OK, if this *is* true, then I need a new place for my shop, since I'm losing it. I need a new place to live. Obviously, the place I am living in is falling apart. I need something new.' I remember thinking, 'I want a brand-new clean apartment.' I don't know why I didn't ask for a mansion, but an apartment seemed more in my range at that moment. I also said, 'While you're at it, I need a new husband.' I thought to myself, 'I want my man from Montana, the man I always dream about.' I remember stopping myself, saying, 'Oh, I'm not ready for him yet. I don't deserve him yet.' So instead, I stated what I felt I deserved in a man. (Can you see how the beliefs of a person limit them?)

From the Seventh Plane of Existence, I was shown how to reach down into the bubble of energy that was my life and stir the energy, simultaneously commanding the changes I wanted.

Once I had finished manifesting, I was back in my body, reflecting upon the strange occurrences of the night.

The next morning I was at home when the phone rang. It was a man named John who owned the only metaphysical store in Idaho Falls. He said to me, 'Vianna, I'm moving my shop. I need someone to move in with me at the new location to help pay the rent. Do you want to move in?'

This was the spark for a series of events that validated the manifestation of the night before. Within two weeks I had moved into a brand-new apartment, moved my shop and met my next husband. I had filed for divorce as soon as I had seen the deepest, darkest secret of the man I was with.

That afternoon I reflected on my existence. The realization that I had created my problems was a bitter pill to swallow. The ability to see truth in people had shaken me. I went up to God and said, 'Why did you do this to me? Why do I have to learn from this experience?' And I received the message, *'Oh, Vianna, Christ could see the truth in people and he loved them anyway.'* I said, 'Well, I don't want this unconditional love stuff, because that's way too much responsibility.' God seemed to smile and was silent.

In time I came to see that truth is what it is and people are just what they are. The ability to see the truth about someone and still love them the way they are is the true meaning of unconditional love.

I had asked God to show me truth and I had met truth. I had met the Law of Truth; it had come into my living room. It had come in the form of faces and balls of formless energy. It had shown me how to see *truth*.

That was my first experience with the Laws of the planes of existence. What I am about to share with you is what I have learned about the seven planes of existence since that time.

16

THE SEVEN PLANES OF EXISTENCE

The seven planes of existence provide us with a conceptual vehicle for understanding how and why the world works on the physical and spiritual levels, and how this relates to us. They show us how to understand the concept of the Creator of All That Is. It is through the Creator of All That Is that we learn how to create physical healing, how to progress spiritually and how to find enlightenment.

The seven planes of existence are divided into degrees. They are not dimensions. There are, however, trillions and trillions of dimensions on the Sixth Plane of Existence, through the Law of Time.

Each plane is subject to its own conditions, rules, laws and commitments, but once understood, all of the planes have the ability to heal. We respect all of the planes and those who have accomplished great works of healing with them. However, the objective of this book is to teach how to access healing abilities from the Seventh Plane of Existence by using the unconditional love of the Creator of All That Is. Through the Creator of All That Is, instant healing, instant accountability and instant results are created. When healing is done from the Seventh Plane, we are under no obligation from the contracts and conditions that govern the first six planes of existence.

It is often necessary to clear ourselves from oaths, vows, rules or ancestral commitments from the first six planes of existence. As we explore these planes in the following pages, we will reveal and clear many of these beliefs and commitments, some of which we may not know we have.

The Creator of All That Is exists everywhere. The energy of Creation exists everywhere. It is all around us. It is what we are. It is what you are. You *are* the seven planes of existence.

THE FIRST PLANE OF EXISTENCE

The First Plane of Existence consists of all non-organic material on this Earth, all the elements that make up this Earth in its raw form and all the atoms on the periodic table before they start to bind to carbon bases. It is the minerals, the crystals, the soil and the rocks. It consists of every piece of Earth, from the smallest crystal to the largest mountain, in non-organic form. Every minute of every day, we work with the First Plane of Existence.

Each plane represents physical and emotional aspects of us. If there is perfect balance, there is perfect health. The less we are able to absorb minerals, the greater the imbalance with the First Plane of Existence and the higher the risk of developing mineral-deficient related diseases such as arthritis and osteoporosis. If our body lacks minerals, there will also be a lack of emotional support and structure in our life.

People who work exclusively on the First Plane of Existence are sometimes called *alchemists* and have the spiritual knowledge of transmutation of minerals from one form to another. The ability to move objects or to bend spoons with the electromagnetic power of the mind is also held on this level, in a marriage with the Sixth Plane.

When a healer uses minerals they are using this plane of existence. Crystal healers use this plane of existence. The use of crystals requires time and energy, and if the facilitator isn't trained correctly, a part of their life force will be taken to do the healing. However, there is a mineral for every sickness, as every plane of existence can be used for healing.

THE SECOND PLANE OF EXISTENCE

The Second Plane of Existence consists of organic material – vitamins, plants, trees, fairies and elementals. The molecular structure of this plane contains a carbon molecule and, therefore, is organic matter. Minerals are non-organic and vitamins are organic; both are essential for life to occur.

Vitamins symbolically give us the feeling of being loved. If they are missing or the body is not absorbing them, it can become out of balance with the Second Plane of Existence. This results in the feeling of a lack of love in the body.

Yeast, fungus and bacteria also reside on this plane. Yeast and bacteria occur naturally in the body and are neither good nor bad. However, it is important that they are balanced. The human body craves what it needs. If a person is low on carbohydrates (sugars), then they are low on energy and will crave them. To experience harmony with the Second Plane of Existence, the body must be in balance.

We live in harmony with the Second Plane of Existence. Plants and humans have developed a symbiotic relationship. Plants use humans to propagate and spread themselves and are, in turn, indispensable to human survival. They perform the miracle of photosynthesis, the sacred creation of blessed sunlight into pure energy for us to consume. We thrive on this energy and plant seeds in the earth to begin the cycle anew.

Plants are highly evolved; they live from light and minerals and, on the whole, use no other living organic material. All plant beings have their own consciousness. Along with the earth and air spirits, plants act out the sacred dance of interconnection between the First and Third Planes of Existence. They transmigrate the life force for the animals to utilize.

Plants and trees are some of the most evolved and sacred of God's creatures. In the cycle of birth and death, they gather nutrients through their roots from Mother Earth and continue to return the same nutrients long after they die. They follow nature's sacred cycle and only compete to live, not destroy. While only consuming sunlight, air and soil to sustain themselves, they provide nourishment and shelter for other living beings.

HARVESTING PLANTS

Love, joy, happiness and respect are the keys to truly understanding plants and trees. When using them to heal, whether they are home grown or wild crafted, we should remember to harvest them with respect.

When you want to harvest plants, speak to them by going up out of your space, connecting to the Creative Force and, through the Creator of All That Is, expressing your need and asking their permission to harvest them. They should speak back to you and direct you to the plant that will best suit the intended use. As you harvest the plant, be connected to the Creator, go back to the time the plant was a seed and pour love and blessing into that seed, and then envision it growing into its present form with this love. This will give the plant more potency.

BLESSING FOOD

When buying herbs, vitamins or food, ask Creator of All That Is if they are for your highest good. We can determine this by connecting to the Creator while holding the product, simply asking if the potency is correct.

Once the substance has passed the test, it should be blessed before use to ensure maximum potency, effectiveness and quality. Since everything has a consciousness and we absorb this essence when we consume it, we need to bless all the food we eat! If these substances have not been treated with the respect they deserve, the benefits will be reduced. Genetically altered food, especially corn, has a consciousness that is perhaps not for our benefit. If there is a question about the provenance of the food, go back and bless it from its origin.

Healers using this plane of existence understand how to use herbs and vitamins in order to achieve health. They understand how to balance the alkaline in the body with food to achieve health.

Every plane has its rules and regulations. Healing from this plane takes persistent use and requires time to take effect. Healers working with this plane require extensive knowledge of plants and reactions to medicines. Without this knowledge, there is a risk to the client. However, as with the minerals of the First Plane, there is an organic combination of plants for every illness.

NATURE SPIRITS

The Second Plane of Existence is the first plane that demonstrates the ability to enjoy life, emotions and feelings. This is the plane where co-existence and survival between planes begins.

There are living organisms connected to the trees and plants. Plants release fragrances to repel bad insects and fragrances to attract beneficial ones for pollination. Plants and trees also have spirits that guard them. These are the fairy spirits and elementals that reside on the Second Plane. Even if fairies are not a part of your belief system, the more that you are in a Theta state, the greater the possibility that you will be able to see these kinds of energies with the naked eye.

The energies of the Second Plane are unique and joyful spirits, though some are just merely curious. They are like yet unlike humans, with their own inconsistencies and passions. Use proper discernment in working with the energies of the fairies because they are incredibly powerful beings and they do not process thought in the same way as humans. They are mischievous and extremely curious and love to annoy us as much as they love to help us.

If we invoke and use the energy of elementals directly from the Second Plane in a manifestation, they will demand something in return for that manifestation. Elementals are sometimes afraid of us and will not reveal themselves because they see us as predators. However, there are water spirits that are the life force of the streams and bodies of water that have their own spirits that will talk to you.

People who work exclusively on this level are sometimes called *wizards*.

THE THIRD PLANE OF EXISTENCE

The Third Plane of Existence is where animals and humans exist. It is the plane of life that has mobility, that exists from eating plants or other animals that co-exist here. This is the plane of protein-based molecules, carbon-based structures and amino acid-based chains. These organic compounds are the basis of life on this plane.

Complex beings, such as humans, have an imagination, great problem-solving abilities and the power to ask the question 'Why?' We often think that we are more evolved than the First and the Second Planes. Perhaps this is because we have an ego, an instinct that was given to us in order to allow us to survive and achieve.

We are actually walking miracles! We learn to manipulate our body, to use our brain, to walk, talk and control our limbs, and have the ability to act upon our thoughts, ideas and dreams. A man imagines a building and he can build it.

It is on this level that we have the challenge of being governed by emotions, instinctual desires and passions, and of being human in a physical world. The Third Plane is the ground where we learn how to control our body, our thoughts and our feelings. This is the plane of imagination, problem-solving, of fight or flight.

You may think that you're physically on the Third Plane of Existence, but you actually exist on all of the seven planes of existence. In reality, humans are from another plane. We are children of the Fifth Plane and seem to have some conscious recollection of this. In fact, many religions are based upon this thought. This explains why we believe that we are 'children of God', because we have a spirit father and mother on the Fifth Plane who call themselves gods.

Because the Third Plane of Existence is the school of Fifth-Plane energies, we are divine in nature and can easily be taught to use a Seventh-Plane force. In fact, in order to graduate from the Third Plane, the human 'student' must learn how to use the Seventh Plane of Existence. Many of the people here on Earth are actually masters from the Fifth Plane who have come here to help their human Third-Plane students/children come home to the Fifth Plane.

If you often feel as though you do not belong here on Earth, that Earth is too harsh, that its people are cruel, and you feel incredibly homesick and miss your spiritual family, you may be a Fifth-Plane master. If you know you have incredible abilities and a strong connection to the Creator, you may be a master waking up to help the Earth. The masters of the Fifth Plane that have come here can easily remember how to direct their mind. All of the high Fifth-Plane masters use the Seventh Plane to create.

Healers on the Third Plane of Existence are governed by time. They often get caught up in the drama of this plane and believe that some things are incurable because of group consciousness. They also often get drawn into a Fifth-Plane energy of good and evil (dualism) instead of a Seventh-Plane energy of love and 'All That Is'.

We live on the illusion of the Third Plane of Existence. Here we have created programmes, thought forms and collective consciousness. Ego, another of our creations, exists on this plane. However, one of the great qualities of this plane is the gift of passion and the experiencing of emotions.

It is through the removal and replacement of belief systems and the addition of *feelings* that we gain an opening to the vibrations of the other planes of existence. It is then that we are released from karmic influences. The more beliefs that are changed, the faster we are able to access the other planes.

Remember, because we are made of minerals and organic material, we're still connected to the other planes.

The component of this plane is proteins. If there is weakness on this plane, proteins are deficient and the structure of the body is deficient. If the body lacks proteins, it will also lack emotional nurturing. However, there is an amino acid for every sickness.

It is on the Third and Fifth Planes of Existence that galactic visitations occur.

Wayward spirits (*see Chapter 20*) reside between the Third and Fourth Planes of Existence.

THE FOURTH PLANE OF EXISTENCE

The Fourth Plane of Existence is the realm of the spirit, where people exist after death and where our ancestors go in waiting. This is what some people would consider the 'spirit world'. Contrary to popular belief and superstition, spirits can still feel, touch, smell, hear and see. They can still eat food and they still have to give themselves nutrition. This world is simply of a higher vibration, where the molecules are moving faster than in the Third Plane. Since no plane is really 'solid', they are all simply different combinations of energy, vibration and light. This is the plane where we learn to master the spirit, or what we perceive as the spiritual aspect of creation.

The Fourth Plane is not governed by time. What may seem like 100 years to you is only a few seconds to Fourth-Plane consciousness. The spirits that exist on the Fourth Plane achieve much learning and new heights of development. Many highly evolved guides come from this plane. Many Goddess-worshipping religions are based here. This is the plane where we find the spiritual energy of the animal spirits and the shape-shifters that native cultures speak of.

OATHS, PROBLEMS AND OBLIGATIONS OF THE FOURTH PLANE

Healers such as shamans and medicine men often use spirits and their ancestors to aid them in healing. Together with spirits and herbs, they are able to achieve many great things. However, healers who understand the specific healing energy of this plane are restricted by the obligations of consciousness that exist there. Some of these Fourth-Plane healers may be restricted by obligations of suffering and oaths and vows that they cannot heal themselves. If this is the circumstance, they must go through the 'Little Death', where they may actually die and come back.

There may also be the consciousness that a disease must be 'taken on' in order to heal it. This is fine for the shaman who knows how to take on and transform the illness to get rid of it later, but many people who have genetically or energetically inherited this ability have forgotten how to get rid of the illness after they have taken it on.

Healers on this plane may be caught up in dualism, the belief that there is an eternal battle between good and evil, and may separate the two opposites that make one, that of Mother Earth and Father Sky.

In summary:

- People using this plane to heal believe that healers cannot heal themselves. This is the plane of exchanging one thing for another, taking a person's sickness upon yourself in order to get rid of it.
- Healers connected to Fourth-Plane energies have a programme that it is wrong to directly accept money for healing sessions. Only gifts are acceptable face to face.
- The obligation of this plane is self-sacrifice and that one must suffer to learn to overcome the negative beliefs of our ancestors.
- It is on the Fourth Plane of Existence that we learn about initiations. There are beliefs on this plane that say a person has to come close to death or 'believe' that they must die to learn more. There is the belief that to master the plane that they are on, they must dance with death or die the 'Little Death' of initiation.
- Spirits on the Fourth and Fifth Plane of Existence have a tendency to be misleading and often make the healer believe they are more special than anyone else. The healer will walk around expecting others to recognize that they have no ego and yet expecting to be honoured, worshipped or feared. One can get a false sense of power from this plane.

WAYWARD SPIRITS

Sometimes when a spirit passes from this Earth they get trapped between the Third and Fourth Plane, afraid to go to the light of the Creator of All That Is:

- These can be spirits who simply do not believe in the light.
- These can be spirits who have committed suicide and had traumatic deaths.
- These can be Native Americans who have died and are afraid to go to the light because they are afraid they will become the light.

These are all wayward spirits and even though they are trapped on the Fourth Plane for a moment in time, it may seem like hundreds of years to us. They can simply be sent to the Creator's light by using a simple wayward spirit exercise (*see Chapter 20*).

FOURTH-PLANE BELIEF PROGRAMMES

Energy test or:

'I have to suffer to learn.'
'I learn the hard way.'
'I am expected to suffer.'
'The more I suffer, the closer I become to God.'
'I have to go through a death door or die to grow spiritually.'

Replace with:

'I learn without suffering,'
'I learn from the Creator.'
'I learn with ease and freedom.'
'I know the definition of dedication from the Creator of All That Is.'
'I am always connected to the Creator of All That Is.'
'I grow spiritually through the Creator of All That Is.'

THE FIFTH PLANE OF EXISTENCE

The Fifth Plane of Existence is divided into degrees; hundreds if you were to count. This is the plane of the ultimate in dualism. The lower degrees of the Fifth Plane are where the negative entities abide. The higher degrees are where the Councils of the Twelve are held. There is a Council of Twelve for every soul family. You may even be part of these councils. Their members are enlightened masters who have evolved past the Third and Fourth Planes and sit together in conferences using their knowledge to help create other worlds. These masters are now being born into this reality in order to change the energy on the Third Plane of Existence.

There are also angels on this plane that have never touched the Earth and have always been on this plane. These angels of light go forth to touch and assist all creatures of the universe.

On this plane there also reside groups of special spirits that come in to assist in healing operations (psychic surgery) when an intuitive person calls them in. We have a spiritual father and mother on the Fifth Plane as well. This is also where the astral plane is.

Understand that the negative degrees of this plane are not mixed with the positive degrees, such as the angels, the Councils of Twelve, our soul families, the masters, our heavenly father or our heavenly mother. The masters, such as Buddha and Christ, are beings that have transcended both a physical and spiritual body. Even though the Fifth Plane of Existence has such enlightened beings, in the lower levels of this plane, *ego* still resides.

People who channel angels and prophets are tapping into this plane of existence. This is the level of the lower gods and goddesses, guardian angels, angels, guides and demons. Each time you connect with these beings, this plane is simultaneously opened to you.

When connected with, the spirits of this plane act as mediators between humans and the Creator. These beings inadvertently interject their own opinions into the information, however, and this can be confusing to the person receiving the messages. One should learn from this plane, but not get swept up in the drama of the battle of *good against evil*, of *ultimate dualism*, or get bogged down by the opinions of the beings of this level.

People who do get swept up in the drama of this plane tend to bring in the belief of 'the end of the world' or other drama-based information, which is still based on sin, fear, doubt and guilt. Healers that work with this plane often read emotions, fears and aggression versus the *Highest Truth of the Seventh Plane*. Remember, while unconditional love is of the highest vibration in the universe, fear is of the lowest vibration.

CONNECTING WITH THE FIFTH PLANE

If you connect to the Fifth Plane of Existence and ask for help from the spiritual energies that reside there, such as angels and ascended masters, you become obliged to follow the rules of this plane. According to the illusion set down in this plane, there must be a 'trade' between the healer and God. However, if you go to Seventh Plane of Existence and ask the same question, the Creator of All That Is may send an angel from the Fifth Plane to do the job, but in this instance you are not bound by the rules of the Fifth Plane.

Also, if you're working with a Fifth-Plane consciousness, be aware that your ego may interfere with your judgement. Then you'll refuse to look at the possibility of not being right. You'll refuse to rethink your decisions; you'll refuse to work on yourself, assuming it is someone else's fault. The Fifth Plane can give you an exaggerated sense of self and make you feel that you have to prove you're right. You pick up group consciousness fears and try to force your importance onto everybody else. You may get false information that you are the only one who has a special power, the only one who has the key to a specific bit of knowledge or the only one allowed to bring it back to Earth.

When you receive information from any spirit, go up and verify it with the Creator of All That Is, because beings on this level have their own opinions. On the Seventh Plane, all information is available to those who ask. The Creator will always help you. Each plane has its own version of truth, but the Seventh Plane is the Highest Truth. What before appeared to be a mountain becomes a small matter when you use the Seventh Plane.

The masters from the Fifth Plane that are here on Earth know that in order to help those from the Third Plane they must relearn how to use the Seventh Plane. At some point in time, they remember their mission:

1. They must teach their students how to use the Seventh Plane and clear their limitations.
2. They must teach their students how to have discipline in their own thoughts and how to tap into All That Is.

Fifth-Plane beings that are not born into the Third Plane can only hold Third-Plane energies for three days, because it is difficult to lower their higher vibration to match the vibration of the Third Plane. It is much easier to be born into a lower vibration and to rise to the remembered higher vibration. This is why the masters are incarnated into this world at this time. Unlike Third-Plane children, they are born with 'knowingness' and will remember all that they need to know in order to bring the Earth to graduation.

FIFTH-PLANE HEALING

Healers using Fifth-Plane energy are bound by the 'rules' and will often heal with a sacrifice of energy, for instance:

'I must be punished.'
'It's selfish to heal myself.'
'I will trade my eyes in order to get the gift of sight.'
'I will sacrifice my life for your life.'
'I have to die to get close to God.'

'I must prove my love to God.'
'I must battle evil all the time.'

Many healers are consumed by the Fifth-Plane drama that is going on and fail to realize that the Creator of All That Is has created *everything* of the All That Is. They find themselves caught up in competition and feeling jealous of others because they are tapping into a lower Fifth-Plane energy.

When healers attempt to tap into the Fifth Plane, they first tap into the boundaries of the Third Plane. They don't realize that these boundaries were only put there in order for them to move above them and go back to the Fifth Plane.

Examples of these boundaries are:

'I am mortal.'
'I have limits.'
'I must prove myself.'
'You have to suffer.'
'You are separate.'

FIFTH-PLANE PROGRAMMES, VOWS OR COMMITMENTS

The history level of belief work may be connected to the Fifth Plane of Existence and many programmes of vows or commitments from another place and time may come into play here. Test yourself or your client for the following vows or commitments and instil the replacement shown.

For the first energy test, investigate for the programme of:

'I have vows or commitments that keep me bound to a plane.'

If the test is positive, investigate what the vows or commitments are. They may include the following:

Power
Energy test for:

'I have to give of my body to gain power.'
'I am afraid to own my power.'

Replace with:

'I understand the Creator of All That Is' definition from the Seventh Plane of power.'

'I understand what it *feels like* to know and have my power because my power is the Creator.'

'I am empowered.'

Love for Another
Energy test for:

'I can love someone and be a healer.'

'I can be loyal to God and be with a mate at the same time.'

'I understand the definition from the Creator of All That Is from the Seventh Plane of being a healer.'

'I understand what it *feels like* to know love.'

'I know what love is.'

'I know when to be in love.'

'I know how to live my daily life with love.'

'I know the perspective of the Creator of All That Is of love.'

'I know it is possible to be in love.'

'I understand what it *feels like* to have love and still love the Creator of All That Is.'

Sacrifice
Energy test for:

'I have to "sacrifice" one of my senses to get close to the Creator of All That Is.'

Replace with:

'I am always connected to the Creator of All That Is.'

Suffering
Energy test for:

'I have to suffer to get close to the Creator of All That Is.'

Replace with:

'I know how to live without creating suffering.'

Proving Love
Energy test for:

'I have to die to prove my love to the Creator of All That Is or to please the Creator.'

Replace with:

'The Creator of All That Is loves me unconditionally.'

The Battle with Evil
Energy test for:

'I have to battle evil.'

Replace with:

'I'm impervious to evil.'
'I understand what it *feels like* to be impervious to evil.'
'I know how to be impervious to evil.'

Taking on the Disease
Energy test for:

'I must have the disease to heal it.'

Replace with:

'The Creator of All That Is is the healer, and I am the witness.'

God is the Healer
Energy test for:

'Only men/women can heal.'

Replace with:

'The Creator of All That Is is the healer, and I am the witness.'

Celibate for God
Energy test for:

'I have to be celibate to be close to Creator of All That Is.'

Replace with:

'I can be loved by God and still have a partner.'

Being Alone
Energy test for:

'I have to be alone in order to be close to Creator of All That Is.'

Replace with:

'I am close to the Creator of All That Is always.'

Destruction
Energy test for:

'The world is heading for complete destruction.'

Replace with:

'I am always safe in the Creator of All That Is.'
'I understand what it feels to live without fear of destruction.'

Healing and Money
Energy test for:

'It is impossible to do healing work if I have money.'

Replace with:

'The abundance of the Creator of All That Is is limitless.'
'I understand what it *feels like* to be fairly paid for my time.'

Trade
Energy test for:

'I traded my gifts of healing, of sight, knowing, hearing, etc., away in order to help someone or to learn.'
'I have to give of my body to gain spiritual power.'

Replace with:

'The gift of healing is mine through the Creator of All That Is.'
'All trades are finished and over. I claim my gifts.'
'I understand what it *feels like* to be the witness as the Creator of All That Is heals.'
'The Creator of All That Is is my spiritual power.'

Vows Preventing Other Intuitive Abilities Being Accessed
Energy test for:

'I have to be dead to connect to the Creator of All That Is.'

Replace with:

'My connection to the Creator has no limits.'

Energy test for:

'I have to suffer to be with the Creator of All That Is.'

Replace with:

'I can be with the Creator of All That Is without suffering.'

Energy test for:

'I have to suffer to grow spiritually.'

Replace with:

'I can grow without having to suffer.'
'I know how to grow without suffering.'

Energy test for:

'I have to die and return to grow spiritually.'

Replace with:

'I can always grow spiritually without dying.'

So now you can understand how we are connected to the first five planes. We are part mineral, part of the plant kingdom because we consume it, part of the animal kingdom because we have a body, part of the spirit realm because we have a spirit, and part of the Fifth Plane. And because we live under the universal laws, we are connected to the Sixth Plane too.

THE SIXTH PLANE OF EXISTENCE

The Sixth Plane of Existence is the Laws. There are Laws that govern our universe, our galaxy, our solar system, the Earth and even us. There are Laws that govern the Fifth Plane, the Fourth Plane, the Third, the Second and the First. It is because of these Laws that there is an imaginary division between the different planes of existence. I say 'imaginary' because they truly exist altogether. When I say 'Laws', I mean the real Laws, the Law of Magnetism, the Law of Electricity, the Law of Truth, the Law of Nature and the Law of Compassion.

Each Law is a huge consciousness that has a smaller consciousness connected to it. They all have a spirit-like essence, a living, moving consciousness. You can invite a Law to speak to you, but it is up to that Law whether it would like to accept the invitation. Tesla channelled the Law of Magnetics and the Law of Electricity. One should always speak with these beings through the Seventh Plane of Existence.

Healers that use the Sixth Plane will heal with tones, geometrical shapes, numbers and light. Any time tones, colours, numbers, magnetism, sacred geometry, the Earth's magnetic grid, astrology and numerology are used in healing, a healer is tapping into the Laws of the Sixth Plane of Existence. Here there is the knowledge of tones that balance the body perfectly, the knowledge of the tone to change any virus in its vibration. The philosophy on the Sixth Plane is, 'If it's broken, fix it.' Often these healers get caught up in explanations and often exude an enormous amount of energy. They often become blunt in their truth and are easily irritated by themselves and others in their quest for truth.

To hold this and other types of 'Law vibration' for long periods of time is hard on the human body. It takes much persistence and practice to hold these kinds of energy. This is the level of *pure truth* and accountability.

Healers using the Sixth Plane of Existence realize that they are living in an illusion and that they are directing their own illusion. They know they no longer need to punish themselves in order to grow and progress. On this plane, the battle between good and evil is eliminated and replaced by pure truth. People who work exclusively on this level are sometimes called *mystics*.

The Laws are structured and tiered with limitless information:

- Under the Law of Truth comes the Law of Motion, which states, 'Once in motion, always in motion.' Under the Law of Motion is the Law of Free Agency and the Law of Thought ('I think, therefore I am'). Under the Law of Motion comes the Law of Velocity and Law of Cause and Effect. Under the Law of Cause and Effect is the Law of Wisdom, the Law of Action and the Law of Justice. Under the Law of Justice is the Law of Witness or Acceptance.
- Under the Law of Magnetism is the Law of Gravity. Under the Law of Gravity is the Law of Time and the Law of Attraction. Under the Law of Time (sacred geometry is under the Law of Time) is the Law of Dimensions. (Avoid getting caught up in the Law of Dimensions, as there are millions of dimensions.) Under the Law of Dimensions is the Law of Illusion, which keeps you thinking that you're here. Under the Law of Illusion is the Law of DNA. Also under the Law of Time are the Akashic Records or the Hall of Records.
- Under the Law of Vibration is the Law of Energy and under the Law of Energy is the Law of Focus. Under the Law of Focus is the Law of Light, the Law of Tone and the Law of Electricity.
- There is also the Law of Nature, which has Laws under her, such as the Law of Balance. Nature is always changing and improving upon the Law of Life. There is no Law of the Creation of Life, because the true creation is All That Is.
- There is actually a Law of Compassion that has the ability to bend many Laws. Under the Law of Compassion is the Law of Pure Intent, the Law of Patience and Law of Emotion.
- There is no Law of Love. Love is a pure Seventh-Plane energy. *It just is.*

You can see that Laws could be discussed for a very long time. There is so much to learn, because each plane has an enormous amount of information. We are advised to avoid getting caught up in this 'brain candy' and becoming bound to any of the other planes, and to go directly to the *Seventh Plane.* Since each plane has so much information and many levels of truth, many healers get distracted. Brain candy is interesting, but it will distract you from your prime objective. That objective is to achieve an instant connection to the Creator for instant healing, full accountability and the creation of a productive life.

THE SEVENTH PLANE OF EXISTENCE

The Seventh Plane of Existence is the pure energy of Creation; it is all-encompassing. This is the plane of 'It just is'. If a healer uses this plane to heal, healing is instant, because the illness is simply re-created as perfect health. Unlike the other planes, where the healer can be exhausted by the plane's vibration, this plane simply embraces you in love energy while it changes the human vibration to perfection.

In this plane the individual is suddenly aware that they can transform energy easily and effortlessly, and simply create their world. Healers using this energy are raised to perfect health. They can use all the planes without being bound by any oaths and commitments. They will realize thought control and have things manifest in front of them instantly. They can clear the limiting beliefs that bind them to the fear-created paradigm. Some healers are afraid of using this plane, thinking that they are going to God's God, but the Creator says you're just stepping into your birthright as one with All That Is, without separateness.

The Seventh Plane of Existence creates the other planes. This is the place of pure wisdom, of the Creative Force, the essence of pure *love*. This is the place of instant healings, manifestations and the highest truth. When a healer connects to the Seventh Plane and witnesses the Creator heal, healing is simply done.

To reach an understanding of the Seventh Plane, one must first realize that the first six levels of existence are only illusions created by the powers of each level. Know that the power and the pure truth is the Creator. Instead of fixing a problem, you just change it. The individual grasps that the world is an illusion and is able to take action on every level.

Healers working on this level achieve instant healing, but only with respect to the client's free agency. Beliefs may be blocking them from an instant healing. With the Seventh-Plane energy, you are consciously aware of every choice. You don't waste time on little idol things, such as drama, chaos and havoc. Issues are changed without self-criticism. Beliefs can be changed instantly.

Healers who work with the Creator of All That Is can move easily in and, if desired, out of all of the planes of existence. With practice, one can instantly manifest things, teleport and have an absolute energy of joy and love.

Be patient with yourself as you evolve. When evolved to the Seventh Plane, one has absolutely no time for useless anger, resentment, competition or regret. One will have the ability to read thoughts instantly without critical judgement of where a person is. When channelling the Seventh Plane, one realizes that everyone's thoughts are a response to what they themselves project out to the world. They are not only conscious of these thoughts, but they can control and easily create the thoughts they choose to. They project co-operation and how to bring everyone to their best. They are awakened masters.

> The 'road map' that I have suggested you use to get to the Seventh Plane lowers the veil of the first six planes of existence.

WELCOME TO THE SEVENTH PLANE OF EXISTENCE

It gets easier and easier to connect to the Seventh Plane when there are fewer negative thoughts occupying space in your brain. Clearing out negative thoughts and programmes on all four levels that keep you bound to the other planes will allow you to maintain a *conscious* connection to the Seventh Plane of Existence *all* the time. The memory and consciousness of all the planes is within you.

When you first go into a Theta state you may initially only reach a high Fifth-Plane energy. This is because of genetic programmes. Your resentments and anger may also prevent you from going up to the Seventh Plane at first. Also, you may never have known that there was a Seventh Plane. Your ancestors may have never been allowed to reach that far because they were confined by the group consciousness of their time.

It is not uncommon for you to think that you've already made it to the Seventh Plane when you haven't, because a high Fifth-Plane energy is filled with lots of love. If you think you're at the Seventh Plane and you're seeing people, angels, kings or queens, then you're not on the Seventh Plane. You're home in the Fifth Plane, which is a great place to visit. You can also heal from there.

Sometimes when you think you've reached the Seventh Plane you will receive an answer that says, 'Go to a higher plane.' You then think that there is something beyond the Seventh Plane, but there isn't. In reality you have yet to get there. So keep going.

It is not uncommon for you to feel discouraged when you feel that you're not reaching the Seventh Plane. However, the more beliefs that you clear, the more you will realize that the Seventh Plane has always been there for you. You are a part of it. Clear your resentments until you are where you want to be.

Also, remember that as long as you go into a Theta brainwave you can witness healing from any plane of existence. Every plane heals. If you're falling ill, you're probably not doing healings from the Seventh Plane.

The illness is an indicator of this and is a sign of imbalance, too much resentment and anger at yourself and others. Remember, this could also be genetic. The point is that now we have a way to clear it. The Seventh Plane doesn't heal or fix things, it simply creates another reality. Until we can access this power in purity, we won't be allowed to use it. So just clear your resentments and keep practising the work.

The more you practise going to the Seventh Plane, the faster you can get there. It may seem as if you only just went up and now you're back! You are going to the nucleus of All That Is. It just is. In this place there is absolute peace, knowingness, contentment, support, nurturing and endless possibility.

THE STRUCTURE OF LIFE OF THE PLANES

The human body is made up of five different compounds: lipids, carbohydrates, proteins, ATP or energy and nucleic acid, which is DNA. These are what make up a living organism. They make you what you are. They are the staff of life that connect you to the other planes.

As mentioned earlier, if they are lacking in the body, there will be a lack in other areas of life as follows:

Lack of:	Will create:
First Plane: Minerals	Lack of support
Second Plane: Vitamins	Lack of love
Third Plane: Proteins	Lack of nurturing
Fourth Plane: Carbohydrates	Lack of energy
Fifth Plane: Lipids	Lack of spiritual balance
Sixth Plane: Nucleic Acid	Lack of spiritual structure
Seventh Plane: ATP	Lack of spirit

The First Plane: If you have a lack of minerals in the body, you will have a lack of support on an emotional level and will be prone to diseases which have to do with a lack of support, such as some kinds of arthritis.

The Second Plane: If you have a lack of vitamins, you will have a lack of love on some level. In turn, if you have a lack of love, you will not absorb your vitamins correctly.

The Third Plane: If you have a lack of proteins, you have a lack of nurturing.

The Fourth Plane: If you have a lack of carbohydrates, then there is a lack of energy in your body and you will have weaknesses in the body.

The Fifth Plane: If you have a lack of lipids, you will be without balance in your system. Your hormones will be off-balance. (Hormones keep your body balanced.)

The Sixth Plane: If you have a lack of nucleic acid, you will have a lack of spiritual structure.

The Seventh Plane: If you have a lack of ATP, you will have a lack of spirit, because ATP is the energy that makes the cell function. This is the *pure energy* that is held in the mitochondria. Mitochondria are the essence that we get from our mother's DNA. They hold ATP. The electrical pulses of the energy of ATP are the home of the spirit. The spirit is in the mitochondria, not in the DNA. The DNA is the computer program, the mitochondria the conscious electricity. When people die and energy is seen leaving the body, this is the mitochondria beginning to shut down.

Low spiritual energies may mean that we have too many soul fragments in too many places.

Everything that you consume in the way of food gives you the knowledge of that food. All things that are consumed have their own intelligence. So if you consume food of a low intelligence, or a slave food such as wheat, you can take on that consciousness. Slave food refers to the food that was given to conquered and enslaved people. Bread was given to Native Americans and black slaves; once they were conquered they were given foods they were not accustomed to eating. On the other hand, royalty ate white bread as a luxury. So certain foods were stigmatized. Always remove the group consciousness that stigmatizes foods such as wheat. A balance can be met by using oats, as they have a different consciousness. Always bless your food.

THE EQUATION OF THE PLANES OF EXISTENCE

Healers always use more than one plane of existence at a time. This is called an *equation*. The healer plays an important role in this equation as the witness:

Creator + Person to Be Worked On + Witness = Result

Many people heal using many planes. They do this by mixing the planes together. When doctors perform surgeries, they are performed from the Third Plane of Existence utilizing imagination, problem-solving abilities and physical application. Even though they are acting on the Third Plane, they are using the Law of Cause and Effect from the Sixth Plane of Existence. They are also using anaesthesia and antibiotics from the Second Plane of Existence and surgical equipment made out of materials from the First Plane of Existence.

In the old ways, a person was expected to master one plane at a time. Every time there was advancement – which often came as a near-death experience – one would have to make a giant mental shift, an 'initiation'. Because of the drama held on all of these planes, the initiation could be traumatic. The true purpose of initiation is merely to reward someone for all of their efforts and their conscious actions, as well as to inspire them to progress further and to evolve. In ThetaHealing, we have learned not to be bound to those planes, to free our minds and advance less traumatically. With the belief work, we are able to pass initiations smoothly without having to sacrifice or die for attainment. In fact, the belief work itself is an initiation.

When a person first begins to use the Theta technique they connect to different planes of power and can be uncertain as to which one that they are on. Since all the planes are connected with the Divine, they can sometimes be confusing. The best way to recognize the planes is to connect to and experience them. Always go to the Seventh Plane first so that you are not bound to the commitments of the other planes.

VOWS OR COMMITMENTS TO CLEAR IN ORDER TO UTILIZE THE SEVENTH PLANE

Some of us are kept from using the Seventh Plane by vows that we do not realize we have, such as:

'I have to be dead to connect to God.'
'I have to suffer to be with God.'
'I have to suffer to grow spiritually.'
'I have to die and return to grow spiritually.'

Since you began as a healer, have you gained weight? If you can feel everyone else's life experiences more than you can feel your own, or if you begin to fall apart physically, it may be because these vows and commitments are still in place on some level of your space. They can be on the emotional, physical, mental or spiritual levels.

Think back to how many times you began to develop as a healer, only to begin to lose other things in your life, such as your car, your husband or your wife. This is the issue of 'sacrifice for power'. As you once again connect with the power of the Fifth Plane, you spirit reacts in remembrance of that power, just as it once did. This means that you may be trapped in those commitments from other places and times and will continue to sacrifice to get healing and information.

The goal, obviously, is to be free of these commitments and to have the ability to use every plane of existence without any commitments or obligations to those planes.

Going up to the Creator gives us the ability to flow with all the planes at one time. However, because we are so intertwined with all the lower planes, we sometimes keep commitments and obligations from them and don't go up to the Creator first. We become so used to only using certain levels that we become bound by the rules of those levels.

In another explanation as to how the planes of existence affect us in this reality, we observe an individual who has had an experience in a past life as a person or as a spiritual being who had knowledge of the powers of the Fifth Plane of Existence. In that time and place the person or spirit knew a great many ways to heal, had great powers, had great respect and had the understanding as well as the *experience* of that plane of existence. But now they have transmigrated to a new body with new challenges. They have forgotten some of their former talents, been stripped of some of their old power, and the respect that they once held from others is no more. They are constantly attempting to recapture the remembered elements of power in this place and time, only to find disappointment in the fact that some of these elements must be re-created through initiations in the present. The ascended master is constantly reminded of the limitations of the human body and faced with the collective belief systems of other inhabitants of this existence. For an old soul, this is one of the initiations facing them: the initiation of reconstructing the elements of power in this life and not constantly pining for the past one.

For the old soul to integrate with the Third Plane of Existence, they must not sabotage themselves in attempts to 'check out' of their present situation. They must learn to accept and enjoy the Third Plane, even as they train themselves to pull back the elements of power from the other planes, as well as develop new abilities for this place and time.

PROGRAMMES WITHOUT LIMITS, PLANES WITHOUT BOUNDARIES

When you were raised in your particular family, you were told what to believe. You were expected to believe as your family did, and because your brain works as a computer, you either took what they told you as a programme or you rejected it. From the time you were a small baby you were told that if you touched a hot plate it would burn you. This is a *stop* sign. As a child you agreed that this was a *truth* and so believed it and took it as a programme. Anything held as a belief will be created in this illusion of the Third Plane in the subconscious mind. So in the act of creating programmes, the mind accepts the illusionary Third Plane to be real, like a computer accepting data.

When you remove, replace or instil belief and feeling programmes, you work with all the planes that you currently are connected to and exist in. When these programmes are removed, you are able to use all the planes at once instead of being trapped on one or two, as all the levels can be accessed in concert with one another, and all the manifestations of power can be used simultaneously or separately as they are needed. As your negative programmes are removed and replaced with *programmes without limits*, you may begin to manifest important changes.

What we chase after is the seemingly elusive feeling of being joined to the Creator of All That Is. What we do not recognize is that this is already ours. We can recognize this, however, when we don't have programmes blocking us. Once these programmes are changed, we can live in the present moment of absolute love and see clearly what is really going on with the people around us. Even though we are in a Third Plane of Existence 'body', we can still tap into absolute truth.

It was once thought that the only way to tap into truth or the other planes was to die to move up and advance into them. But now we know that the key to advancing is in *this* space and time, in *this* physical body, to become the master in *this* incarnation. It is important not to get bogged down with our Third Plane of Existence emotional belief systems, or the belief systems of other spirits and energies in and on the first five planes, as well as to understand the powers of the planes and how they pertain to healing.

MANIFESTATIONS OF BELIEF

We are manifestations of what we believe and how we are programmed. Everything we are makes us what we are in our body, in the *now*. What we believe we are, we are. If we have too many negative beliefs, it causes an energy fracture in what we are. In order to fix these energy fractures, the Creator has given us illnesses to make us aware that they exist.

If you're dealing with too much guilt, for example, you will attract bad bacteria. (Most bacteria are good for your body.) If you have too much resentment, you will draw fungi into the body. By the same token, if you feel that you are unworthy, you will draw viruses. Belief work can clear these emotions and vibrations.

When a person is truly unwell, they will always tell you that they are ready to change and will do *anything* to get better. In some instances, however, they go back to their old habits because they don't know how to live without the negative beliefs that hold the disease to them. Some of these feelings are programmes of rejection or programmes of resentment. If the person does not change their beliefs or instil new ones, the cycle of disease starts all over again. For instance, an antibiotic has the correct vibration to heal bacteria. But if you were to do the necessary belief work, you would not draw the bad bacteria to you in the first place.

By observing people, we are beginning to map individual diseases and the beliefs attached to them. There will be a reference map available in the future.

Ask the question, 'What is lacking in this person to draw these diseases? Is it love?' It may be that there are *feelings* that are lacking, feelings that the person has never known.

'I AM SEPARATE'

One thing that allows sickness to come into the body is the programme of 'I am separate'. When your consciousness leaves your body to do a healing on someone, you realize that all things are a part of the All That Is. But when we move back into our space and realize that we have a body of skin and bones, it makes us think that we are separate.

Most of the problems that occur in this existence are caused by illusions. For instance, I have found that many people have the illusion of 'Separation from the Creator' and the illusion that we physically exist in the flesh.

This is why some healers gain weight. In their fear of becoming All That Is, they gain weight to maintain their identity and to stay separate. But when you move your essence 'up' to do healing in the body, you realize that the Creator moves through all things and you're a part of All That Is. This is a wonderful feeling for that moment, but we're programmed to have an *identity*. In order to keep the illusion of individuality, some healers overcompensate when they bring themselves back into their space. They ground to this plane so rigidly that their body gains weight to anchor them to this illusion. This can be an unconscious response on the part of the healer. They have a healer side and a more personal side designed to maintain and own an identity. In fear of losing this identity they build programmes to be separate. This is why when you bring the energy back into your space, you should go down into the Earth and ground out and then bring it back up to the crown chakra. This is training your body to know that you are a part of All That Is.

The idea that life is an illusion is a wonderful concept to believe in, but you must *know* it too. The illusion is that you are separate, but you are not separate from God, you are a spark of God. When you *know* that you can be connected to that energy and still live in a human body, you may realize that you don't even have to eat. You come to know it as a philosophy and then come to the actual *realization of truth* that you don't have to eat.

When you have a realization such as this, you create your own paradigm. Nothing can get in that energy because you are no longer separate. You will not be psychically attacked; you will not vanish into thin air ... unless you want to.

HEALING WITH THE PLANES

As I have told you before, we exist in seven planes of existence. Each of the planes has a cure for every emotion or disease in the body. On the First Plane there is one chemical combination or one mineral combination to heal every disease. On the Second Plane there is one plant or vitamin, or possibly several plants or vitamins, that will act as a cure for every single disease. We live in the plane of proteins, which means there is one amino acid combination that will heal any sickness.

Knowing that you *can* heal on these first three levels, as well as on all the other planes, will explain why you go into a healing crisis. In the process of healing there is a period when you go through all sorts of emotions. So when you are using a herb from the Second Plane, the healing crisis forces you to cleanse the body, but it also forces you to clear out unneeded emotions.

On the Fourth Plane of Existence there are spiritual advisors and a spiritual essence that will heal any sickness in the body. Shamans marry the Fourth and Second Plane, using plants and spiritual energy to heal. The essences of these two planes will usually make you promise to do certain things, which will change your vibration.

On the Fifth Plane of Existence the heavenly fathers and the angels can all heal your body. You may have to trade for the healings or make changes for them, but in the process, they clean up belief systems.

Once connected to the Sixth Plane of Existence, you will hear music and tones. To heal from this plane, vibrations are used.

When it comes down to it, all the planes are about *music* and *light*. All are about *vibration*. Using the correct mineral to heal is all about using the right vibration within the mineral. Using the correct herb to heal means using a herb that has the right vibration. All of these physical things that you consume for healing have the same vibration as the belief work that you do. An antibiotic herb that has the right vibration to heal you from a bacterium, for example, also has the right vibration to heal you from the guilt that draws the bacterium. It is possible to do belief work with every cure from every plane.

RE-CREATING

Prior to teaching a seminar in Seattle, I tripped over my dog's food bowl and took a nasty fall. When my husband Guy brought me into the house, I realized that my knee was dislocated. My first thought was, 'I have to do a seminar! This is *not* going to happen.' So I went up and said, 'No, this isn't here. This did not happen. Go back to the way you were!' My knee went back instantly. That's when I noticed that I had broken my finger. It was pretty obvious, since it was bent off to one side. I put my hand over it because I didn't want to see it. I commanded it to heal. Instantly I was out of pain and was healed. That's Seventh-Plane energy and the way to use it: deny that the situation is happening and create a new one in your life.

When I tell you to go to the Seventh Plane, I tell you to 'discreate' the illness, not to shrink it. This means that you must create the reality that there is no illness, tell the body that it is denied and that there is a new scenario. Witness this. In order for you to do this, however, you have to clear up limiting beliefs that say you can't.

CLEAR YOUR MIND

I have students come to me and say 'I've been working on my beliefs for a year and I'm not completely better yet.' Do you want to know why? They're working on the *wrong beliefs*. They should first work on the beliefs that clear the mind. The belief that heals them might be one tiny little belief out in the auric field of the body. Once they clear their mind, they'll be able to see it and release it. They'll be able to wake up in the morning and be better.

Ask the Creator, 'Which beliefs do I need to clear?' But you may have to ask the right question, for instance, *'Which beliefs do I need to work on to take care of this symptom?'* It is possible that the challenge is twofold in nature. You may get two answers: clear your mind and release a particular belief.

17

'HEALER, HEAL THYSELF'

I know that those of us who heal knew even before we were born that at some time in our lives we would step up and become healers. The question is how to do it most effectively.

In order for you to do effective work on people, it is important that they allow you into their space. Your belief system is also very important, since things can be changed and healed simply with the healer's faith alone. However, it is best if you do feeling work on a person before doing healing, such as downloading the feelings of 'I know what the Creator's love *feels like*' and 'It's possible to be healed' and 'I deserve to be healed'. Once the person has been prepared, they will believe they deserve instant healing and that they don't have to suffer.

In this process, at the moment of healing conception, you will 'discreate' what is in the person's space and create something new. In that moment of discreation and re-creation, you touch the very essence of the Creator. In that moment you will feel an incredible surge of energy. It will surge through your body, into the body of the client, then flow through both of you together and then it will be gone. This is the experience of instant healing. It is as addictive as any drug on the planet. Once you have had it, you will want to experience it all the time.

INSTANT HEALING

Instant healing is the discreation of a belief system, and the energy of that belief, and the creation of a new one. This is when you touch the Seventh Plane and can see actual *creation*.

Since 2003, I have been witnessing more instantaneous healings than ever before. The reason for this is that the more people know how to tap into the belief of instant healing as a group consciousness, the easier it is to do instant healing. The more people that are given the keys to open the doorway to illumination, the stronger all of us will be in healing through the Creator. As we become as *one* in our thoughts and create a group consciousness, we will all experience instant healing.

As healers, we want instantaneous changes, but we fail to recognize all the things that go into making the body what it is. The body is composed of millions of cells. So, when you want instant healing to be performed, you are asking for thousands of cell changes to happen right when you want them to. And all these cells have their own intelligence. Just as we can pick up on the thought processes of people as we walk across a crowded room, so can your cells. What is important is whether or not we accept these thoughts as truth. The projection of healing works in much the same way.

I expect a healing from Creator, but I am not attached to that outcome. If a person heals, they heal. If they don't, they need belief work. If they are being sent psychic surgeons and tones in their healings, they have belief programmes that say they can't heal instantly or that it may take time for them to heal.

When people do not heal instantly, they like to place blame on others and give others the responsibility for their illness. Healers need proper discernment in these matters, knowing that God is the healer and not them. The healer is just the witness of what happens between a person and God. So don't become attached to the outcome of a healing.

Some people are not ready for instant healing and will heal gradually instead. A person's ability to accept healing has a lot to do with them getting better. Look at the person to see where they are coming from in their belief system. If they think they should get better in three to four months, they are saying that they need more time to heal. If they don't believe that they deserve healing, you may need to work on them with regard to their feelings and beliefs before they get better. For instance, you do a healing on someone and command their cells to be completely better, but they go home and are still ill. In this case I would say that the thought form of healing has been interfered with. The person has belief or feeling work to do so their body will be in agreement and then they will heal.

As we have already seen, there are people who want to be healed and people who want to be sick. Some people will come to you in an attempt to get you to carry their illness for them. Some keep an illness because it serves them well, or is their entire life experience. Every one of these people needs the balanced love that comes from the Creator. The healer's role is to be the witness, to be the conduit for love from the Creator but not directly responsible for the healing.

A person may not be able to accept instant healing. It may be that they need to take a vitamin to get better, or even have surgery. But you can prepare them for instant healing.

PREPARING FOR INSTANT HEALING

When you are getting a person ready to experience instant healing you need to teach them what it *feels like* to:

- Forgive others and forgive themselves.
- Have joy.
- Have the Creator's love.
- Be worthy.
- Be able to accept a healing from the time that they were in the womb onward.

All the people that I have seen experience instant healing have shared certain beliefs and feelings:

'I understand what it *feels like* to be worthy of God's love.'
'I understand what it *feels like* to be healthy.'
'I understand what it *feels like* to be loved.'
'I understand what it *feels like* to love myself.'
'I understand what it *feels like* to have joy.'

BELIEF BLOCKS FOR THE HEALER

Energy test yourself for these programmes:

'Healers are evil.' (An ancestral fear.)
'Psychics are evil.'
'I fear healing.'
'I doubt healing.'
'I have boundaries on healing.'
'My healing abilities are blocked.'
'I will be killed for being a healer.'
'I must suffer to be close to God.'

UNDERSTANDING HEALING

PROGRAMMES ABOUT LOVE

When I was a little girl people always disappointed me. I knew that they couldn't love me, because they didn't know how to love anything or to receive love. I realized that I had to love them first and then they could learn to love me. The reason that most people cannot be good to you or to be nice to you is that they do not know *how* to love, or the *feeling* of love.

As a child, I thought that loving people meant seeing only the good parts of them, not the bad. My mind was changed when I saw the truth about people in the Akashic Records and the truth about unconditional love.

We all think that we understand the feeling of love, but many of us do not. So energy test for the programme 'To be loved I have to be needed constantly'. If you test positive for this programme, reaffirm in yourself 'I have balance with love' and 'It is safe to be loved' or 'I love God and God loves me'.

- Energy test to see if you understand the Creator's definition of what it *feels like* to be surrounded by people you love and who love you in return in the highest and best way. Instil, 'Creator of All That Is, it is commanded that I understand what it *feels like* to be surrounded by people that love me.'
- See if you understand the Creator's definition of what it *feels like* to be surrounded by people who are intelligent, uplifting individuals, people that build your spirit and help you soar. In return, you will build them up and help them soar.

If you have become a healer so that everyone will love you, you are in the wrong profession. People come to you for their own reasons. They may come to you because of their sickness, but they really come to learn from you, to learn about the Creator of All That Is. Ask them what you can do for them and then use the healing processes that are needed to help them. Instil:

'I understand the Creator's definition of love.'
'I understand the Creator's definition of love for my human body.'
'I understand what it *feels like* to allow someone to love me.'
'I understand what it *feels like* to have discernment and love.'

If you test no for these programmes, then bring in the feeling and the knowing of love from the Creator on every level – physically, mentally, emotionally and spiritually.

SEE TRUTH – KNOW THAT YOU ARE PROTECTED

When you go into a room and feel the energy in the air, make sure you have proper intuitive discernment. When all of your abilities are developed it will be possible to sense every bacterium in the air and every parasite on the ground. Psychically, I can feel every worm in someone's body. But if I were to let it affect me, I would be frozen and wouldn't be able to function.

Physical senses become very receptive for many psychics, and we can openly feel other people's emotions and thought forms. Ironically, we spend all this time trying to develop our psychic abilities and, when we finally do, we may find another person's thoughts too harsh. So be aware that you can become offended by people but not know why, and you may simply want to get away from them.

You need to be able to recognize these thoughts and energies, yet still be impervious to them. You need to know the truth and still be able to function. Many intuitives create walls of protection because they don't want to feel all the wild energy in a room, or in the world. When they do this they aren't seeing the truth, because it is filtered by the defence shields that they have created. But if you shine your energy out then nothing can touch you. If you radiate the Creator's energy, you can change any energy. You will be totally protected by God and nothing will be offensive to you.

GO UP AND GO OUT

There are old psychic processes that teach that you should stay completely in your own space. This teaching tells you to maintain a 'protection bubble' around yourself at all times and never to leave your space at all. It seems to me that this takes a lot of time and energy and is also fear based. Instead, consider radiating your aura with the essence of love. Let any negative energy that comes your way to simply flow through, around and from you and be changed to love and light to feed you and sent to God's light. When you are connected to the Creator, negative thought forms and psychic attacks will melt as snow in spring to create pure water to wash you clean.

Download the Creator's definition of:

'I am impervious to evil.'
'I am impervious to attack.'
'I am impervious to others' negative thoughts.'
'I know how to see truth.'
'I know what the truth is.'
'I know that I am protected.'
'I know the difference between my thoughts and another's.'
'I shine the Creator's light to the world.'

HEALING ADDICTION

It has been my experience that some people create sickness to get attention, nurturing and love. They become dependent on the healer and are afraid that they will die without them. There have been times when I have considered refusing readings and healings for someone because they expected me to live their life for them. The trick is to give them back their own power, a power that they may never have had.

Endorphins are released into the system of a client each time they experience a reading, and this may be why they come back.

I am careful to honour everyone who comes to be worked on, even when I do not agree with why they came to me.

PROGRAMMES OF PAST FAITH

In the past, religious people were eaten by lions and healers were stoned or burned. If you have the feeling that these may be your past experiences or that they may be genetic memories, energy test for:

'I am wrong to defend myself.'
'To test my faith, I have to die.'
'I have to suffer like Jesus.'
'I have to prove myself to God.'

Replace with:

'It's safe to defend myself.'
'I have proven myself to God.'
'I can believe in Jesus and still defend myself.'
'I know what it *feels like* to be in service to humankind.'

If someone says, 'I'm blocked. I can't do this work,' see if they traded their gift of sight or healing away in order to help someone in another time or place. Go up and command that this past energy be cleared and finished and that they be allowed to receive back their gifts.

PREPARING FOR HEALING

AN EXAMPLE OF PREPARING A MAN FOR HEALING

To help someone heal it is useful to know their background. That will show you what you might be up against. Let's say a man comes to you to be healed. You enter his space and see all the things that are going on in his life. He is 40 years old and has been divorced for a year and has just met and married a young woman of 20. He thinks his ex-wife is cold and insensitive and he has two teenage daughters that he is paying maintenance for. He has a good job and is prosperous and ambitious. The young wife wants a home in the country, and because he loves her, he takes out a mortgage to secure it. The house has lead from old pipes, and the water that comes from the well has been tested for bacteria, but not for heavy metals. What he does not know is that there are trace elements of arsenic and nitrates. The house has a little mould in the walls and has lead paint. But the new couple moves in and in a whirlwind of activity the new wife begins to renovate the house.

The bills begin to mount up between the two wives, past and present. The man becomes very busy at work to generate income to pay all these bills and begins to use coffee to stay awake on the drive from the country home. He complains to a friend that he has no energy and the friend gives him some pills to keep him up. Because he spends so much time at work, the beautiful young wife has an affair with the interior decorator.

After about a month the young wife finds that she truly loves her husband and breaks it off with the decorator. In remorse, she confesses to her husband. Hurt and incensed for a time, he finally decides to forgive her. Unfortunately, the decorator has given our couple the gift of herpes. To add to the problem, one of our hero's daughters becomes pregnant and the ex-wife is incessantly badgering him for money and support. Now unable to sleep, he goes to the doctor to get some sleeping pills.

So! Our hero has heavy metal poisoning, is breathing fungus, uses speed and tranquillizers and has herpes and more stress than the body can take. The body hits overload level, and to control and encapsulate all of these toxins and emotions, it creates a place to put them: cancer in the prostate.

After all this, he comes to you to be healed. He needs help on his perception of his life. First, teach him what it *feels like* to be loved. Maybe he *feels* that anyone he loves will betray him. Teach him that he is worthy of being loved. Teach him what it *feels like* to be healthy, to be in balance. Also, he will have to clean up the heavy metals, the fungi and moulds, not to mention the addictions to drugs. You can witness the Creator heal the person, but if all the other factors are not put into balance, the cancer may return.

AN EXAMPLE OF PREPARING A WOMAN FOR HEALING

A woman comes to you to be healed. You enter her space and see all the things that are going on in her life. She is 40 years old and been divorced for a year from her husband, who has remarried a young woman of 20. She thinks her ex-husband is an insensitive pig and she hates his new wife. She has two teenage daughters that she is almost solely responsible for. She has never had a steady job and now has to keep one. The divorce has given her a large house, but there are still payments on it. The teenage girls have gone wild, so in order to watch them her mother invites herself in, with whom the woman has a love–hate relationship.

She starts work early, works late and begins to use ephedrine to stay awake on the drive from home. She complains to a friend that she has no energy and has gained weight, so the friend gives her some pills to help her out. She works as a secretary at a chemical plant and is exposed to dangerous fumes from time to time. Unfortunately she falls into a rebound love affair at work, only to find out that the man is married. Let's call him Peter.

The woman is hurt and incensed for all time and eternity, and decides to swear off men forever. Unfortunately, Peter has given her a parting gift: chlamydia. To add to the problem, one of her daughters becomes pregnant and it becomes necessary to badger her ex-husband incessantly for money and support. Now unable to sleep, she goes to the doctor to get some antibiotics (for the chlamydia) and sleeping pills.

So! Our heroine has chemical poisoning, uses speed and tranquillizers, has just had chlamydia, has internal hatred and more stress than the body can take. The body hits overload level, and to control and encapsulate all of these toxins and emotions it creates a place to put them: cancer in the ovaries.

After all this, she comes to you to be healed. First we need to teach her what it *feels like* to be loved. Maybe she *feels* that anyone she loves will betray her. Teach her that she is worthy of being loved, what it *feels like* to be healthy, to be in balance, as well as release all the hatred inside. Also, she will have to change her job and stop using the drugs. You may witness the Creator heal the person, but if all the other factors are not put into balance, the cancer may return.

> *It is interesting to note that I have done readings on divorced couples without either ever knowing that the other was seeing me.*

THE NATURE OF HEALERS

Generally speaking, there are two different kinds of healers that I have dealt with in the teaching of this work: those who serve everyone and those who think that if they become a powerful healer everyone will serve *them*. (Both, by the way, are dysfunctional!)

The first type forgets the love of self. They are constantly looking for the lost and lonely soul that needs help. (This can be a full-time job.) They want to help all humanity and cry when others are hurt. They let others walk over them. They are so busy helping others that they set no boundaries. Generally, they don't understand what it *feels like* to love themselves or to know that God loves them. Finally the physical body is affected and they find themselves very alone when they need love. The danger to this type of person is that they may become sick simply in an effort to receive some love.

The other kind of healer is on the other side of the scales. They expect the world to worship and adore them. They have love of self, which is good, only they love themselves too much and forget to love others in the process. This type of person only serves themselves, and wants everyone else to love and serve them. They need to understand what it *feels like* to love another person or love God.

These two basic types of people have the same feeling but with different motivations. There are those who *over*-serve and those who *under*-serve. You may fall into either one of these categories depending on the day and how you feel at the time. Balance is the key. Both types of healer need to meet somewhere on middle ground, in service and in love of humankind, without forgetting their *self*.

18

Death, Initiations and Death Doors

A true intuitive is sensitive to the world around them, particularly the feelings and emotions of others. We are like a canary in a mine shaft: the first to feel the effects of the poisonous influences around us. These influences can be physical or metaphysical; both are hazardous to a sensitive person if they do not learn to release or become impervious to them. In a healing, the emotions and feelings of others can be overwhelming, particularly when someone has been told that they are terminally ill. These emotional reactions to the prospect of death may keep us alive or hasten our demise.

THE WILL TO LIVE ... AND DIE

I am and always have been an advocate for life over death. I have cheated death so many times in my life that I have lost count. It was only after witnessing thousands of healings that I came to realize that some people come to a point where they do not want to be healed. This is one of the cold, hard facts of life. You cannot heal a person who does not want to be healed. The healing will roll off them like water from a duck's back.

If your client will not accept a healing in any area of the body, you will sense it. This is the time to ask them whether or not they truly want to be well. If they do not want to get better, just accept it. Some people who are dying want it that way. You must allow this to be.

Here are two examples of how I learned that it was not me against death in a battle of duality. Death is not the enemy, it is another part of All That Is.

LIVE FOR ANOTHER

I had a very good friend who had cancer. I came to love him very much. He came in for healings on a regular basis when we first started developing the

Theta technique. As I worked with him I could see the changes that were occurring, but I could also feel that he didn't want to be healed. Finally I confronted him with this feeling. This is what he said to me: 'Vianna, I have lived my life and I have been useful. I am in my seventies now and no one wants me anymore. I am tired of this life and I want to go on to something different. The only reason I come for these healings is so that my wife will think that I am making an effort to get well.'

Always make sure you understand the motivation of the person you are working with. You are not at fault if they do not want to be healed. Since healing comes from the Creator and not from you, you must never feel guilty or assume any blame for a person who does not want to be healed.

SHELLY: THE SPARK FOR BELIEF WORK

This story is about courage, the will to live, the will to die and how I learned how to accept death.

I learn something from every person who comes into my office. I have seen many people that have truly impacted my life, but one of those who left a lasting impression was Shelly. Up until the time she came into my life, the mentality that I had was that it was *me against death*. I had almost died myself and I wasn't going to let death take any of my clients, not if I could help it. Death was the enemy until Shelly showed me a different viewpoint.

Shelly was an unusual person. She had three-year-old twin daughters and was a single mother. She had a rare form of genetic cancer that caused both benign and malignant tumours to grow in different parts of her body. In fact, the disease was so rare that the doctors were treating it for free. They were amazed that she was alive at all with all the surgery that she had had and all the tumours that were in her body.

When I first met her she had recently had a tumour removed from her brain. When they had taken it out, it had been necessary for the surgeons to replace part of her skull with a plate made of titanium. Unfortunately, she had a reaction to the plate that caused a staph infection and they had to remove it. They folded the skin over the opening in the skull and told her to be careful and not to bump her head.

Shelly also had so many tumours in her kidneys at that time that the doctors wanted to remove them. I could never understand this because, even though she had all those tumours, her kidneys were still working. The doctors told Shelly that it was not possible to remove her kidneys, though, because she had so many tumours in her lungs. They first had to shrink the tumours in her lungs, so they prescribed new medication that would be administered daily. They told Shelly that it would make her feel so ill that she would be bedridden.

This was all going on when I first met her. We did repeated healings on her during this time, and it must have helped because she was up and about while on the medication. It was amazing to watch her progress.

Shelly was a smoker and I told her repeatedly to quit smoking. She told me, with that dry humour she had, 'Well, Vianna, I like to smoke.' She was a funny little duck!

This was before we had the belief work. In fact, it was Shelly who inspired me to develop the belief work. It was because of my sessions with her that we discovered how to pull a belief.

She would come in for healing from time to time, then she would leave and I wouldn't see her for a while. This went on for quite some time. In between she would travel all over the state and come back to tell me all about it. She told me that she had never realized how many beautiful places that there were in and around Idaho. She took her little girls to Yellowstone Park, Craters of the Moon and other places. She did all this while she was on the experimental medication.

Shelly and her sister knew that my husband, Guy, ran a Native American sweat lodge ceremony. They came to me and wanted to have the experience. Guy agreed. During the ceremony, he had all of Shelly's family and friends individually pray for her. Those of you that know what a 'sweat' is know that it is physically challenging, but Shelly did just fine. Her health was amazing during this time.

Then came the day when she came into my office and I could sense that something had changed. She arrived when I was eating lunch. At the time, I needed to see 20 clients a day to pay my bills, and my daughter Bobbi and I had only a half an hour in which to eat. Shelly often came in for healings at noon, when I was available.

On this particular day, she sat down on the desk and began to talk. She said, 'You know, Vianna, life is like a game of Yatzee.'

I said, 'It is?'

Shelly said, 'Yep. You know, my first husband was a quadriplegic. He was the meanest man I ever knew. I used to play Yatzee with my roommate waiting for him to pass on. I thought it was wrong to leave him because he was a quadriplegic. Finally, I couldn't stand it anymore and I did leave him. You know, my children's father left me when he found out I was pregnant. So I sat there, pregnant with my twins, and I played Yatzee with my roommate. Now I live with my mother and my doctors won't let me work anymore. They tell me I am too sick to work so I sit at home with my mother every night and I play Yatzee.' She looked at me. 'Vianna, I am so tired of playing Yatzee.'

With that she jumped off the table, gave me a hug and walked out of the door. I thought to myself, 'I need to get in a session with her. Something isn't right.'

About two weeks after that I got a phone call at the office.

'Is this Vianna?'

'Yes.'

'Vianna, this is Shelly's sister and she is dying. She gave me a list of people that she wanted to say goodbye to and you are the last person on the list. I only had your first name, so I have been asking for you all over town, and now that I have found you, I want to know, would you like to say goodbye to Shelly?'

Through sobs, I said, 'Yes, of course I want to say goodbye.'

Shelly's sister gave me the directions to her house.

On my way I picked up my daughter Bobbi and my two-year-old granddaughter Jenaleighia (Jena for short), because Bobbi wanted to come along. When we stopped to get gas, Bobbi got out of the car to pump the gas for me. I was alone with little Jenaleighia, who was buckled in the car seat. Jena had started to talk at an early age. Now she piped up from the back seat, saying, 'Whatcha' doin', Grandma?'

I turned around and explained, 'We are going to Shelly's house. We are going to go and do a healing on Shelly.'

Jena asked me, 'Can I help?'

I said, 'Sure you can help.'

Jena closed her eyes and was quiet for so long that I thought that she had gone to sleep. Finally, she opened her eyes and said, 'There! Shelly's better now, all done! All done, Grandma. Shelly's dying.'

I found this strange, and I was shocked that she knew what 'dying' was at two years old.

We followed the directions and found the house where Shelly lay dying. We found out that she was in a morphine-induced coma and, following her instructions, without food and water. Her sister said that if I had been there two days earlier, she would have been awake. She told me how, a few days before, there were motorcycle riders racing up and down the street making a racket. Shelly had asked her sister to help her to the door so that, as they drove by, she could open her robe to flash them. Shelly was a real character!

Bobbi wept uncontrollably and I watched as Jena wiped her tears, saying, 'Don't cry, Momma, it's almost over now.'

It was in that instant that I realized that Shelly didn't want to live. To her, death was not bitter; it was a release.

I sat beside Shelly on the bed and went up out of my space to check on her. I saw her spirit floating above her body. She saw me and said, 'Vianna! Where is the light? I can't find the light!'

I told her, 'It's OK, Shelly, it's right here.' Then I showed her a great pillar of light that led to Creation and said goodbye to her. I had done all that I could for my friend and I left the house in tears.

From that day on, for me, death wasn't a bad thing anymore; death was simply what it was. This didn't help me when I missed someone when they died, but it made me realize that sometimes death was a welcome friend.

It was because of Shelly's life and death, as well as those of many others who passed away, that we started to develop the belief work. I can't tell you how many nights I stayed up crying to myself, praying and wracking my brain, looking for a way to change the way that people with disease felt about themselves and the world around them. Then the belief and feeling work came to us, and I felt that I could make a difference. With this work I could help more people to live. I might not be able to save everyone from death, but I could certainly prepare them for it.

DEATH DOORS

Death doors are opportunities given to us by the Creator to return home. When we are given such an opportunity, we may accept or decline. This choice is given to the higher self and, from there, to the soul. The soul chooses whether or not it will go to God's light.

When a person declines a death door, their life changes and they grow spiritually. They also become more intuitive. With this transition, new guardian angels are appointed to the individual. This is an initiation of evolvement.

A person who has recurring death doors may have negative programmes about death, spiritual growth and the Creator. To change these programmes, use the belief work. Energy test the person and pull and replace any programmes that are not for their highest good.

THE DARK NIGHT OF THE SOUL

The dark night of the soul is a concept from the writings of Saint John of the Cross. These writings were composed in 1547, when Saint John was imprisoned for months on end in a dungeon by his own Christian order because of his beliefs. In the darkness of his cell, all that was left to him was God. This concept – that through great suffering and deprivation, a higher consciousness can be attained that brings the individual closer to God – has now become mainstream in the collective consciousness.

The dark night of the soul experience sounds ominous. Yet many intuitives and people with a spiritual nature seem to experience this phenomenon while on the road to higher consciousness. The reward that comes after the dark night seems to be finding the profound joy of their true nature.

To a person going through the dark night, suffering seems unending. It is a lengthy and profound absence of light and hope. The person feels profoundly alone. They experience great difficulty in their lives and will face their greatest fear. At times, they *create* these great difficulties because this is the only way they know to grow spiritually.

In most instances, the dark night of the soul only occurs once in a lifetime. It is used as a karmic growth tool for the soul.

Energy test for:

'I am in a dark night of the soul.'

Replace with:

'I understand what it *feels like* to be completely accepted by God.'
'I know *how* to be completely accepted by God.'
'I know *how* to live my daily life completely accepted by God.'
'I know the perspective of being completely accepted by God through the Creator of All That Is.'
'I know it is possible to be completely accepted by God.'

Energy test for:

'I know *how* to evolve spiritually without creating suffering.'
'I have to "sacrifice" one of my senses to get close to the Creator of All That Is.'

Replace with:

'I am always connected to the Creator of All That Is.'

Energy test for:

'I have to suffer to get close to the Creator of All That Is.'

Replace with:

'I know how to live without suffering.'

Energy test for:

'I have to die to prove my love to the Creator of All That Is.'

Replace with:

'The Creator of All That Is loves me unconditionally.'

19

GUARDIAN ANGELS

A guardian angel is a spirit assigned to a particular person to protect and guide them. The concept of angels goes back as far as recorded history, to the Sumerians, and throughout history has been a pervading belief system. The belief that the Creator sends a spirit to watch every individual was common in ancient Greek philosophy and the Old Testament, although it is referred to somewhat non-specifically. In the New Testament, Jesus says that children are protected by guardian angels:

'Never despise one of these little ones; I tell you, they have their guardian angels in heaven, who look continually on the face of my Heavenly Father.'

I've had so many experiences with guardian angels that they are almost too numerous to count. A good example happened years ago, in a reading I had with a woman. I could sense that she had a strong female spirit watching over her. When I went into her space I was told that this spirit was her guardian angel. The guardian angel said to me, 'Tell her that I held her when her son died.' I told the woman this and she broke down in tears. When she had composed herself, she told me her son had died years before and she had been so upset and so overshadowed with grief that she had gone to her room and wept uncontrollably. While she was weeping, she felt as if someone's arms were around her, gently rocking her back and forth. From that moment on she knew that she was not alone and began to feel better.

I am always amazed at the incredible support that guardian angels bring us. I have found them with every person, in every religion and nationality known to humankind. Every person has at least two guardian angels, one male and one female. I have found there are two to four guardian angels per person. Every single one of these guardian angels has a particular name and a particular energy. I have learned that they are not always compatible and may disagree with each other. However, I have come to realize that they only have the best interests of the person at heart.

Guardian angels never leave a person unless they refuse to go through a death door. At that point, as already mentioned, their life will change and evolve, and new guardian angels may be appointed for them.

Guardian angels may also leave when a person goes through the dark night of the soul, at which time the angels may be replaced with another set who will be there to walk the person's life with them.

Spirit guides, on the other hand, can be a different kind of angel from the Fourth or Fifth Plane and can come and leave as they are needed. People can have many, many guides at one time. Any time there are more than 20 guides in a person's space, this is a sign that they are on the verge of a major transition or starting their life's purpose.

If at any time you see a guardian angel or guide who appears to be two years old, you are probably observing a child waiting to come into that person's life. They will appear on the left side of the person (your right side if you are facing them). They may be children or grandchildren that are soon to be born to them or to someone who is close to them.

All of the information that you receive from a guardian angel should be cleared with the Creator, because angels and spirit guides have their own opinions as to what is right or wrong. Even though they have your best interests at heart, pure truth is only with the Creator.

If you ask for specific help and healing from angels, you become obliged to follow the rules of the Fifth Plane of Existence. According to the illusion set down in this plane, there must be a trade for healing. However, if you go to the Seventh Plane of Existence and ask for the same thing, the Creator of All That Is may send an angel from the Fifth Plane to do the job and in this instance, you are not bound by any of the rules of the Fifth Plane. This is not to detract from angels. To experience the energy of an angel is a magnificent event.

THE PRINCIPLES OF GUARDIAN ANGELS

- Guardian angels may appear as human spirits, ancestors, animal totems, spirits, fairies or nature spirits.
- A person usually has two to four guardian angels.
- A spirit guide is different from a guardian angel. A spirit guide will move in and out of a person's world, whereas a guardian angel will stay until a death door opens or the person undergoes the dark night

of the soul. At this time, a more elevated guardian angel comes to assist. This shows us that we are never alone in our space and have assistance at all times.

• The guardian angel technique (*see below*) will enable you to contact a person's guardian angels (or your own) and also show you when children are coming into their life. The spirit will have the appearance of a baby or young person on the left side of the individual being read.

• To tell the difference between guardian angels and wayward spirits (*see Chapter 20*), simply check out what you have seen and heard with the Creator. Guardian angels will be happy for you to ask God to verify information, whereas wayward spirits will throw a fit. Bear in mind that both guardian angels and other spirits have their opinions, and these opinions may not be pure truth.

CONTACTING GUARDIAN ANGELS

The guardian angel technique is an introduction to the spirit world that is all around us. The most important aspect of this technique is that it reveals the difference between the voices of the Creator of All That Is and those of lesser spirits. It also shows that we are not alone in our own spirit realm, or even in our own electromagnetic auric field.

This exercise also gives you the opportunity to practise discerning the different energies in a reading and recognizing the difference between the voices and energies of spirits that are positive and negative.

To see and speak with guardian angels you are going to use the same steps as before, with minor variations:

THE GUARDIAN ANGEL TECHNIQUE

1. Ask permission to see the person's guardian angels.

2. Centre yourself in your heart and visualize going down into Mother Earth, which is a part of All That Is.

3. Visualize bringing up energy through your feet, opening each chakra to the crown chakra. In a beautiful ball of light, go out to the universe.

4. Go beyond the universe, past the white lights, past the dark light, past the white light, past the jelly-like substance that is the Laws, into a pearly iridescent white light, into the Seventh Plane of Existence.

5. State the following: *'Creator of All That Is, it is commanded to see and speak with [name of person]'s guardian angels at this time. Thank you! It is done. It is done. It is done.'*

6. Move your consciousness over the head of the client, into their crown chakra and down into their space.

7. Once you are in their space, look over their shoulders. You may see balls of light. Then command to see faces and ask the guardian angels' names and their purpose.

8. Tell the person what you have seen and heard.

9. As soon as the process is finished, rinse yourself off and put yourself back into your space. Go into the Earth, pull the Earth energy up through all your chakras to your crown chakra and make an energy break.

Θ *You can go up and see your own guardian angels using these same steps by sitting in front of a mirror and going into Theta.*

20

WAYWARDS, THE FALLEN, POSSESSION, PSYCHIC HOOKS, CURSES AND IMPLANTS

It is important that we have a clear perception of the concept of evil. This concept is related to fear and hatred. It was an important milestone in the evolution of the consciousness of humankind. It is used as an excuse to explain floods, famine, earthquakes and natural disasters. As it relates to human behaviour, it was created to explain behaviour or acts that at some time in history became morally unacceptable. At some point in time the idea of duality was formed – an ultimate good and an ultimate evil battling for supremacy in nature as well as inside humankind.

With the belief work it is possible to find and release programmes of evil that may be creating friction in our existence. Remember, evil is fed by fear. When we talk of good and evil we go back to the childhood programmes of 'I am afraid'. I don't think we should actually use the terms 'good' and 'evil'; it is a question of *balance*. Whenever there is a battle or controversy, there is an imbalance, and whenever there is an imbalance there is likely to be a *physical* disability. So we need to create balance in our life.

Energy test for:

'I have to fight constantly against the evil forces of the universe.'
'I am opposed by evil.'
'I have to fight the forces of evil.'
'I know how to be safe.'

Use the belief work and replace with:

'I can choose to battle evil.'
'I am impervious to evil.'
'I am safe.'
'The truth is pure balance.'

Or use the programme that best suits your vibration.

Removal and replacement of these programmes will show the truth about good and evil.

In the modern metaphysical world there has also been a great deal of hysteria about negative spirits, aliens, implants, psychic attack, reptilian energies and the like, and to some people, these represent evil. Replace these programmes with 'I am safe' from these influences.

In ThetaHealing it is also taught that these aspects are nothing compared to the purity of the Creator of All That Is. The Seventh Plane is beyond the concept of 'good' or 'evil' and there you will find only the purity of the Creator.

Energy test for:

'Life is boring without evil to fight against.'

Replace with:

'I am entertained by life.'

WAYWARDS

When you begin to experience the Theta state, you start going into a dream state. In this dream state, you start to be receptive to energies that were formerly invisible to you. As their psychic abilities open, many people become receptive to metaphysical and spiritual energies. These can show themselves as spirits. Some of these spirits are good and some aren't.

Some of these spirits are called waywards. This is a word that I learned from a wonderful woman named Barbara Hughs, who lived not far from me in Idaho. Barbara was a retired schoolteacher who spent much of her life pulling discontented spirits off people, alongside her other healing work. She explained to me that a wayward is a spirit that has left the body at death and doesn't know where to go. Barbara was a gifted healer and has now gone to the same light of God that she sent all those waywards to.

HOW WAYWARDS GET LOST

Our lives are built on an invisible grid system, a grid system of the universe. This follows natural laws such as the rotation of the Earth and gravity. It is so real that even NASA waits for a 'window' before sending ships into space, so they can arrive at the destination they are seeking.

There are openings in the lattice work of this grid system leading back to the Creator; these are the death doors. We are totally connected to the

Creator at all times. However, we are granted many death doors and each of us has our own pattern of opportunity to use them. Once again we are talking about the free will of the spirit.

A death door becomes a 'window' when the soul is committed to go to the Creator. A window stays open for about nine days after the death of a person. When they miss this window of light, the grid system closes again and they are trapped by the magnetic pull of the Earth, so their spirits are left to walk this planet. They return to the places on Earth that they were the most accustomed to, or to the people they loved, or to their place of death. They do not live there as such, but are in a holding pattern for a space of time between the Third and Fourth Planes of Existence.

The Creator has not abandoned these individuals; in good time, they do find their way to the home of the Creator. The Creator's conception of time is totally different from our own, however. What to us may feel like a long time, from God's perspective may be a very short time.

In the meantime, lost, searching for God's light, these spirits will use our radiances as beacons to guide them to the path to return to God. This is why waywards may be attracted to you. In some instances they will attach themselves to you and feed off your energy. This may cause difficulties.

A person who has carried a wayward spirit with them for a period of time may have a physical illness caused by the wayward draining energy from them. As soon as the wayward is gone, the symptoms can completely vanish. There can be more than one wayward attached to a person. A person who uses drugs or is an alcoholic has more openings in their auric field and tends to invite in more wayward spirits.

Don't converse with wayward spirits, since they may be manipulative, angry and crazed. Send them to God's light. Once they go to the light, they will go through a filtering process that releases all negative emotions and programmes from them, so when they come back from the Creator, they will be balanced once again and then it is permissible to call upon and speak with them.

If you do decide to speak to a spirit, never permit it to enter your body. Allowing a spirit into your body can be detrimental to you mentally and physically, causing obesity and mental illness. You may permit the spirit to enter your auric field, around your body, in order to speak to it, but never ever permit spirits to enter or 'take over' your body.

Disembodied spirits are so common that they are a feature of many religious practices. Some Native American teachings maintain that if a spirit goes to the light it loses its identity and becomes part of the light. So in some instances a spirit might feel the need to stay on Earth to keep its identity. There are also native spirits that choose to stay and become guardian spirits for sacred sites.

People who commit suicide are often afraid to go to the Creator's light, fearing punishment in hell. In fear, the spirit rejects the Creator's light. People who have died tragically, in murders or freak accidents for example, may also become so disoriented or so upset at how they died that they miss their opening to the light.

True love can also cause a spirit to miss an opening in order to stay close to its loved one. The spirit may feel that person cannot make it without them. This makes grief a heavy feeling in the house. If you send a lonely spirit like this to the Creator's light, it will most likely return, only uplifted and with less grief.

There is a law that states that wayward spirits must listen once a healer calls on the Creator. So use your connection to God's light to send wayward spirits to the Creator of All That Is of the Seventh Plane as follows:

THE PROCESS FOR WAYWARD SPIRITS

1. Centre yourself in your heart and visualize going down into Mother Earth, which is a part of All That Is.

2. Visualize bringing up energy through your feet, opening each chakra to the crown chakra. In a beautiful ball of light, go out to the universe.

3. Go beyond the universe, past the white lights, past the dark light, past the white light, past the jelly-like substance that is the Laws, into a pearly iridescent white light, into the Seventh Plane of Existence.

4. Make the command: *'Creator of All That Is, it is commanded that all wayward spirits around [person's name] be sent to God's light to be transformed. Thank you! It is done. It is done. It is done.'*

5. Move over to the person's crown. Witness the wayward spirits being sent to the Creator's light using your connection or the client's connection to Source. Be sure you follow them all the way to the Creator's light, as they will attempt to escape.

6. As soon as the process is finished, rinse yourself off and put yourself back into your space. Go into the Earth, pull Earth energy up through all your chakras to your crown chakra and make an energy break.

THE FALLEN

There is another group of spirits called the Fallen. These are different from waywards. They are spirits and entities that shouldn't be here on Earth. They are a little bit nastier than regular waywards.

You can send the Fallen to the Creator's light in a similar way to the waywards. Once you use the Creator to do this, it is one of the Laws of Nature that they must obey the command.

THE PROCESS FOR RELEASING THE FALLEN

1. Centre yourself in your heart and visualize going down into Mother Earth, which is a part of All That Is.

2. Visualize bringing up energy through your feet, opening each chakra to the crown chakra. In a beautiful ball of light, go out to the universe.

3. Go beyond the universe, past the white lights, past the dark light, past the white light, past the jelly-like substance that is the Laws, into a pearly iridescent white light, into the Seventh Plane of Existence.

4. Make the command: *'Creator of All That Is, It is commanded that I hear and be given the name of the entity. Thank you! It is done. It is done. It is done.'*

5. Move over to the person's crown.

6. Find the fallen spirit or entity in or around the body and, using its name, command that it be sent to God's light.

7. Witness it being sent to God's light using your, or the other person's, connection to the Creator. The spirit must obey universal Law.

8. As soon as you have finished, rinse yourself off. Put yourself back into your space, ground to Mother Earth, pull Earth energy up through all your chakras to your crown chakra and make an energy break.

POSSESSION

I never gave much thought to possession until I experienced it directly. This experience came at a psychic fayre in Twin Falls, Idaho. The room didn't have any booths to separate the readings for privacy, so we all did our readings in the open. There were seven psychics doing readings at once. Friends, acquaintances and my ex-husband Blake were in the room watching the goings-on. Two of these people were young Mormon missionaries, relatives of Blake. The room was hot and stuffy and I thought of going home. But since we had travelled such a long way, I decided to stay.

All of a sudden, there was a commotion from a lady who was getting a reading. She started to speak with different voices and roll around on the floor like in the movie *The Exorcist*. Well, I have never seen so many people disappear that quickly in my life, including the missionaries! Everyone in the place ran away in terror, leaving me alone to deal with the situation!

As I walked over to help, the woman's eyes rolled back in her head, her face and body convulsed and she uttered foul words. Touching her shoulder, I knew that she was possessed and I instinctively put myself into a Theta state to send the waywards to God's light. Surprisingly, she had more than one spirit in her body. In fact she had the most spirits that I had ever seen up until then. Eventually all of the waywards that were possessing her were sent to God's light. A little while after that she was fine.

Many people who have been diagnosed with mental problems are prone to possession, so it is good to check for spirit possession as you do your medical intuitive sweep of the body.

Another type of possession is by the entity 'created' by the abuse of drugs or alcohol (*see page 190*). Removal of these entities from the afflicted person may help in their recovery.

The spirit that is possessing the body of the person must obey the command that you send to it when you are connected to the Creator of All That Is.

THE PROCESS FOR POSSESSION

1. Centre yourself in your heart and visualize going down into Mother Earth, which is a part of All That Is.

2. Visualize bringing up energy through your feet, opening each chakra to the crown chakra. In a beautiful ball of light, go out to the universe.

3. Go beyond the universe, past the white lights, past the dark light, past the white light, past the jelly-like substance that is the Laws, into a pearly iridescent white light, into the Seventh Plane of Existence.

4. Make the command: *'Creator of All That Is, it is commanded to know the name of this spirit in the body of [person's name]. Thank you! It is done. It is done. It is done.'*

5. Move your consciousness over to the person's space.

6. Name the spirit and command that it be pushed down through the feet of the client.

7. Command that the spirit be sent to the Creator's light using your or the client's connection to the light. Witness the spirit going all the way to the Creator's light.

8. As soon as the process is finished, rinse yourself off and put yourself back into your space. Go into the Earth, pull Earth energy up through all your chakras to your crown chakra and make an energy break.

ENTITY ENERGY IN DRUG ABUSE

Drug addiction and alcoholism can leave people open to entities. The addiction causes a spiritual energy drain that opens the person to parasitic energy and an entity is able to intrude into the weakened 'space', or aura, of the person.

All the drug-addicted people that I have experienced psychically have had strange entities attached to them. Each drug seems to have an entity peculiar to it and intuitively it looks the same from person to person.

To help an addicted client, move their serotonin level (*see page 266*) as the Creator directs and go into their space to see if anything needs to be detached and sent to God's light. If they are on drugs, an entity will be attached to them. These spiritual entities will attach themselves to the addicted person, gain a hold on their mind and whisper to them the words that keep them addicted to the substance. They must be sent to God's light to ease the suffering of the addicted person and give them a chance at recovery.

These are what some of the forms of addictive energy may look like:

- A heroin spirit looks like a shrivelled old man with hollow eyes.
- A marijuana spirit looks like a brown-haired woman.
- A cocaine spirit looks like a white-blonde haired woman with electric blue eyes. Her energy will be flowing around the addictive person.
- A crystal methamphetamine spirit looks like a white-blonde haired woman with blank holes for eyes.
- Each type of alcohol has a different spiritual energy attached to it. These look different from one type of alcohol to another. Why do you think they call it 'spirits'?

GHOST IMPRINTS

With ghost imprints, the energy of living matter projects memories upon places and objects. The energy is picked up from emotional events or collected from the people that used the places or articles. Furniture, jewellery, pictures and musical instruments may all develop ghost imprints. There are places, too, such as houses, sacred sites, battlefields, boats and cemeteries, that have their own personality due to ghost imprints. These can all 'come alive' as a result of interaction with biological life forms. Hence, a house becomes 'haunted' in and of itself, regardless of any spirits that inhabit it. It will creak and groan and move parts of its own volition, for example opening windows and doors. So, a 'haunting' in a house may not be caused by spirits but rather by the collected sentience of the house itself.

Land, meanwhile, may retain imprints of the events that took place there. So people may see 'visions' of war and carnage while standing on an old battlefield, for example. These are imprints left over from the strong emotions experienced by the people involved in the conflict. These imprints create a vortex, or opening, in space and time, and it is then possible to see the past events.

To experience a ghost imprint that is instilled in a physical object, simply touch or hold the article in question. Open your psychic senses to permit the energy from the article in your hands to flow through you. This technique is an empathic reading and you may see, feel, touch and taste sensations from the object, as well as hear it speak to you.

Spirits and waywards can also attach themselves to inanimate objects such as tarot cards, because we give energy to the cards, which then become like a living entity with a sentience all their own. Remember to clear special articles, i.e. crystals, wands, ceremonial objects and antiques, with the crystal light of the Creator.

CLEARING AND BELIEF WORK ON NON-ORGANIC MATERIAL

Because objects can hold memories, emotions and feelings, and sometimes gain a sentience or consciousness of their own, with belief work you can pull curses off a piece of land or you can return soul fragments that the land has lost, just as you would with a person. You can even teach your house what it *feels like* to be a home.

CLEARING AND BELIEF WORK ON NON-ORGANIC MATERIAL PROCESS

Variations of this exercise can be used with any object.

1. Ground and centre yourself in your heart and visualize going down into the centre of Mother Earth, which is a part of All That Is.

2. Visualize bringing energy up through your feet, into your body and up through all the chakras.

3. Go up through your crown chakra, raise and project your consciousness out past the stars, the universe. Go beyond the universe, past the white lights, past the dark light, past the white light, past the jelly-like substance that is the Laws, into a pearly iridescent white light, into the Seventh Plane of Existence.

4. Gather unconditional love, make the command: *'Creator of All That Is, it is commanded to teach this home the feeling of [whatever you want to teach the house], in the highest and best way. Thank you! It is done. It is done. It is done.'*

5. When you have finished, rinse yourself off in a stream of the water or light of the Creator of All That Is. Enter your body through your crown chakra. Send your consciousness down into the centre of Mother Earth to ground yourself, then pull the energy of Mother Earth up into yourself and make an energy break.

PSYCHIC HOOKS

A 'psychic hook' can arise when there is an emotional attachment to another person. When you feel sympathy, concern or pity towards another person, an energetic bond can be created between you. Since thoughts and emotions have a physical substance, this energy is willingly released to help another. In a scientific test conducted at a hospital it was proven that there was energy going from a mother to her child when the child was lying ill. The mother was feeding the child part of her soul energy of her own free will. Hatred, anger and obsessive love can also create psychic hooks. All these kinds of emotional attachment, of both a negative and positive nature, can be unfavourable to the overall well-being of an individual.

There are varying degrees of depth to a psychic hook. With an extremely intense emotional attachment, a soul fragment can be lost to another person. A soul fragment, as already mentioned, is a tiny piece of our essential life force. It is essential to reclaim soul fragments that have been lost.

PSYCHIC HOOKS AND THE HEALER

It is important for a healer to have a certain degree of objectivity regarding their client. If they begin to feel uncontrolled pity for all of the people they work with, too much energy is expended. There will soon come a time when they are used up and can no longer help anyone. As a healer, the idea is to have balanced compassion, not uncontrolled pity, for the people187you will be associated with. These individuals are creating their own lives. True compassion is doing what is best for a person, rather than feeding on their emotional drama. But even the best of us can get a psychic hook. Here's how to break them:

BREAKING PSYCHIC HOOKS

1. Centre yourself in your heart and visualize going down into Mother Earth, which is a part of All That Is.
2. Visualize bringing up energy through your feet, opening each chakra to the crown chakra. In a beautiful ball of light, go out to the universe.

3. Go beyond the universe, past the white lights, past the dark light, past the white light, past the jelly-like substance that is the Laws, into a pearly iridescent white light, into the Seventh Plane of Existence.

4. Make the command: *'Creator of All That Is, it is commanded that this psychic hook that is attached through [person's name] be released, sent to God's light and transformed into love and light. Thank you! It is done. It is done. It is done.'*

5. Witness the psychic hook being released and sent to God's light.

6. When the process has finished, rinse yourself off and put yourself back into your space. Go into the Earth, pull Earth energy up through all your chakras to your crown chakra and make an energy break.

PSYCHIC ATTACK

Psychic attacks originate from the thought forms of other people. We naturally discard most thought forms that are sent to us, except from those people who are close to us, but some thought forms may constitute a psychic attack. In many instances the person sending the attack has no idea they are causing pain to someone who is intuitive. If a family member is the one directing the thoughts, the person's auric field will not protect them as effectively, since people are more open to thought forms that are familiar.

Wayward spirits and otherworldly beings may also be the cause of psychic attacks. Command that the wayward spirit be sent to God's light of Creation (*see page 187*).

If you suspect you are the victim of a psychic attack, energy test for:

'I have to battle evil all the time.'

Replace with:

'I am impervious to evil.'

Θ *As you become acquainted with the Seventh Plane of Existence and the Creator of All That Is, it will become impossible to be affected by psychic energy attacks.*

THE PSYCHIC ATTACK PROCESS

1. Centre yourself in your heart and visualize going down into Mother Earth, which is a part of All That Is.

2. Visualize bringing up energy through your feet, opening each chakra to the crown chakra. In a beautiful ball of light, go out to the universe.

3. Go beyond the universe, past the white lights, past the dark light, past the white light, past the jelly-like substance that is the Laws, into a pearly iridescent white light, into the Seventh Plane of Existence.

4. Make the command: *'Creator of All That Is, it is commanded that all psychic attacks be automatically sent to God's light. Thank you! It is done. It is done. It is done.'*

5. Witness the psychic attack being sent to the Creator's light.

6. As soon as the process is finished, rinse yourself off and put yourself back into your space. Go into the Earth, pull Earth energy up through all your chakras to your crown chakra and make an energy break.

OATHS, VOWS AND CURSES

Ever since I started doing readings, people have come to me carrying curses of all kinds – Mexican curses, generational curses, spells, and so on. Some people know they have them, others do not.

One of the most profound experiences I have ever had with a curse came from a nice lady who came to me with a unique problem. She was physically unwell and everything was falling apart around her. She had just met her mother-in-law and had accidentally insulted her. I could see that her mother-in-law had put a curse on her because she did not like her. When I went into her space I could see that it was a voodoo curse that had been put on her. It was in the form of a tall, looming black man who was slowly choking the life from her. This was when I didn't know the best way to deal with curses. Instinctively, I brought light from God and sent it through every cell of her body and pushed the curse out of her feet. Then I gathered it up and sent it back to the practitioner who had cast it in the first place. I gave the lady a hug goodbye, confident that it had gone.

A few minutes later I felt a strange heavy sensation beginning to come up my arms. It was the curse, and I knew that the voodoo practitioner had sent it back to me. It was so strong that it started to come up into my body and I could feel it beginning to take me over. In a panic I commanded that it be sent to the light of God and that it to be so through the Creator. It slowly receded from my arms until it was gone. Then I felt a presence in my space. It was the black man in the curse. He had come through God's light and had returned. He thanked me for freeing him from his bondage. The lady recovered from her illness and her troubles stopped.

This is how I learned that you should never send a curse back to the sender. This only causes a war. Send the curse to God's light and use the belief work to give the person the programme of 'I am impervious to curses'.

GENERATIONAL CURSES

One type of curse is a genetic or generational curse. This is a curse that has been handed down from an ancestor who has knowingly or unknowingly accepted that thought form. The person afflicted with the curse will have experienced repetitive difficulties where things seem to attack them. Some examples of this are accidents, insanity, alcoholism and continuous bad luck.

A good example of this comes from the Bible when Moses addressed the Israelites when they were preparing to enter the Promised Land. He told the new generation that they could not enter unless they dealt with their own personal sins and also the sins of their fathers. The account can be found in Leviticus 26:39-42:

'Those of you who are left will waste away in the lands of their enemies because of their sins; also because of their fathers' sins they will waste away. But if they will confess their sins and the sins of their fathers, their treachery against me and their hostility toward me, which made me hostile toward them so that I sent them into the land of their enemies, then when their uncircumcised hearts are humbled and they pay for their sin, I will remember my covenant with Jacob and my covenant with Isaac and my covenant with Abraham, and I will remember the land.'

CAST CURSES

As well as ancestral curses being passed down, a curse can be 'cast' at a person in the present time. However, it is only when the person has guilt, fear or a negative programme that they will receive and accept a curse.

Casting curses seems to be a practice as old as civilization, perhaps older. Here are some interesting examples.

Greek and Roman Curses

Greek and Roman curses were somewhat formal and official. Called *katadesmoi* by the Greeks and *tabulae defixiones* by the Romans, they were written on lead tablets or other materials and generally invoked a spirit (a deity, a demon or one of the dead) to help them to accomplish their goal. These writings were put in a place considered effective for their activation, such as a tomb, cemetery, sacred spring or well. In the text of the *katadesmoi* and *defixiones*, the petitioner uttered a prayer or formula that the enemy would suffer injury in some specific way, along with the reason for casting the curse, such as theft or loss of respect. The Romans, Etruscans and Greeks in Italy all practised this custom. Fortunately for us, they buried the curses so well that today we have a body of curse inscriptions to tell us how they practised their magical incantations.

Voodoo Curses

Voodoo is a religion that originally came from Africa to Haiti, and then went from Haiti to New Orleans. Two hundred years ago, it was transformed and enhanced by a very powerful practitioner. In New Orleans it became what is called Gris-Gris. With Gris-Gris, the practitioner can send a curse or a blessing upon a person in numerous ways. In most cases voodoo is a respected philosophy; very few practise it in a negative way.

BLESSINGS

The opposite of a curse is a blessing. These aspects are two opposing forces of the pervading belief in duality: the forces of 'light' (good) against those of 'darkness' (evil). Both begin as condensed thought forms. The big difference between the two is that blessings can be supported by the Creator, whereas curses have only the support of elements that are less than divine.

OATHS AND VOWS

An oath is either a promise or a statement of fact calling upon something or someone that the oath-maker considers sacred, usually a god, as a witness to the binding nature and the truth of the statement as fact. To swear by or swear on something is to take an oath, such as when a person swears on the Bible in court. An oath is more profound than a promise and binds the person on a deeper level.

There is confusion between oaths and other statements or promises. For instance, the current Olympic oath is really a pledge and not properly an oath, since there is only a 'promise' and no appeal to a sacred witness. Oaths are also confused with vows, but really a vow is a special kind of oath. Oaths and vows can be generational as well, and even though they may have been created for a positive reason, may cause the person difficulties in the here and now.

A self-proclaimed oath or vow spoken by an individual may have far-reaching effects, similar to the effects experienced in a curse. As you investigate the cause of a client's challenge, use energy testing to find if they have taken an oath and if it is causing them problems.

THE CURSES COMMAND PROCESS

1. Centre yourself in your heart and visualize going down into Mother Earth, which is a part of All That Is.

2. Visualize bringing up energy through your feet, opening each chakra to the crown chakra. In a beautiful ball of light, go out to the universe.

3. Go beyond the universe, past the white lights, past the dark light, past the white light, past the jelly-like substance that is the Laws, into a pearly iridescent white light, into the Seventh Plane of Existence.

4. Make the command: *'Creator of All That Is, it is commanded that the curse or vow that [person's name] has be removed from them, from all that they are. It is completed and no longer needed. Thank you! It is done. It is done. It is done.'*

5. Move your consciousness over into their space.

6. Go into the person's space and tell the curse that it is completed and finished. Witness the energy of the curse being removed from all four belief levels, from the physical DNA outward to their auric field. Witness the curse being pushed out through their feet. Gather it up and send it to God's light, never to return, to be transformed into love and light.

7. As soon as you have finished, rinse yourself off. Put yourself back into your space. Go into the Earth, pull Earth energy up through all your chakras to your crown chakra and make an energy break.

8. Use belief and feeling work on the person.

IMPLANTS

Ten per cent of Americans claim to have had UFO experiences of one kind or another. The conception of implants comes from the modern UFO craze that began in 1947. In the 1960s reports of alien abductions began to surface. Implants seem to have begun in 1967 with a woman who described a tiny spiked ball that had supposedly been inserted up her nose. Soon such devices began to proliferate, one of which survived and was thoroughly investigated by the Centre for UFO Studies in the late 1980s. It had supposedly been implanted by extraterrestrial abductors and was later dislodged when the abductee caught a cold and blew his nose. It proved to be a common ball bearing!

Nowadays abductees sometimes discover unexplained objects in their body during routine X-rays and MRI scans. Neither the doctors nor the abductees are able to explain how these objects got there. Doctors do know that a foreign object can enter the body unnoticed during a fall, however, or while running barefoot, or as a splinter from an impacting object. They may then be surrounded by a membrane, like several of the recovered 'implants'.

In his book *Confirmation,* Whitley Strieber describes several implants, including one removed from his own external ear by a physician. It turned out to be collagen, the substance from which cartilage is formed. Strieber admits that the 'hard evidence' provided by implants is inconclusive. 'I hope this book will not cause a rush to judgment,' he writes, 'with skeptics trying to prove that evidence so far retrieved is worthless while UFO believers conclude that it is proof. Both approaches are a waste of time, because the conclusive evidence has not yet been gathered.'

Numerous implants have, however, been removed and studied. Since 1994 several alleged implants have been surgically recovered from such extremities as toe, hand, shin, external ear, etc., but all are different. One looks like a shard of glass, another a triangular piece of metal, still another a carbon fibre, and so on. The implants are generally no more than an inch (3cm) long and a sixteenth of an inch (1mm) in thickness. One implant is wire-shaped and under an electron microscope seems to have a complex structure containing many different layers. Tests have shown that it is composed of a variety of metals and alloys.

In the early years of my practice, people came to me with all kinds of attachments and implants that they felt were inside them. Many of these people worked for the government. I was not so much interested in what the implants were or where they came from as in helping the person to overcome their challenge with them.

Because of what I learned about this and other aspects of the paranormal, ThetaHealing in the present time teaches the use of belief work to remove programmes of being a victim to aliens and other negative, fearful aspects. These programmes should be replaced with 'I am impervious to evil', 'I am impervious to aliens', and so on. Then the person can use the feeling work to instil from the Creator any feelings that they do not have or understand that will assist them in overcoming implants or aliens.

One experience that I had with implants stands out from all the rest. A wonderful woman would periodically come in for healing because she was being attacked by aliens and plagued with implants. I would strengthen her aura and send the 'implant' to God's light. This was well before the belief work, so I did not have this means to work with. She would be left alone for a while, only to have the difficulties return.

One day, she came in for a healing and my husband Guy was there. He was sceptical about implants and this was something that I wanted him to learn. I asked the lady if it would be alright if he attended the healing and she said that he could. So I had him come into the healing room to see a 'real' implant. On this occasion the lady had an implant in her arm. It moved up and down her arm and I wanted Guy to witness this with me.

Guy put his hand on the lady's arm where the implant was. It moved under her skin and this alarmed him. He stepped back and said, 'What the hell is it?!' Then she held her arm out and we all could see the implant move under her skin. This experience pushed my husband's belief system to the limit.

I commanded that the implant be sent to the light of God, never to return, which it did. After that, it was gone.

I do not know what it was in her arm and I don't care. What I do know is that you could touch it, see it and watch it move. The important thing was that the lady believed that I could help. Eventually she stopped having these experiences with such intensity, and when the belief work came to us, she used it to empower herself. In ThetaHealing today, we do not have an opinion as to the validity of implants or alien energies, we simply help a person heal.

Implants are generally found in people who are working in government positions or believe they have been abducted. If they believe it, then it is real. However, many people who are very intuitive are mistaking viruses and bacteria in their bodies for 'implants'.

If in the process of a reading you hear the Creator tell you the person has an implant, first ask them if they have a breast, tooth or surgical implant. Do not command all implants to be removed from a person until you have explored to see if they have a pacemaker or steel pins or have had any number of different types of surgery where foreign matter is left in the body.

If the implants are not of this type, don't over-analyze what they actually are, where they came from or have the person relive the experience of the implantation or alien abduction. Simply empower them with the belief and feeling work.

When someone has difficulties with alien abduction memories, the programmes are generally held on the history level. Muscle test for the memories, and if they exist, resolve them with the belief work. If they are not real, then the person has made them up to cover up real experiences of trauma. Remember also that a virus is an alien invader in every cell. Psychically and microscopically, it may look like a robot. If asked, God may agree that a virus looks like an alien invader. So, when a person is telling you that they have an alien problem, they may not be wrong, it is only their perception of the 'alien' that is. As an intuitive healer, you will need to listen to the person until they can work out whatever the fear is and find the real problem. If you follow their 'brain candy,' you will find the greatest fear. Listen to their belief system. They will choose which beliefs they want to keep or to drop. The Creator of All That Is can change anything, so don't live in fear, just go up and change whatever is needed. Convince the person that freedom from abduction and fears of aliens is reached through the Creator.

THE PROCESS FOR IMPLANTS

1. Centre yourself in your heart and visualize going down into Mother Earth, which is a part of All That Is.

2. Visualize bringing up energy through your feet, opening each chakra to the crown chakra. In a beautiful ball of light, go out to the universe.

3. Go beyond the universe, past the white lights, past the dark light, past the white light, past the jelly-like substance that is the Laws, into a pearly iridescent white light, into the Seventh Plane of Existence.

4. Make the command: *'Creator of All That Is, it is commanded that I know and hear the tone that destroys this implant that is in [person's name]. Thank you! It is done. It is done. It is done.'*

5. Move over to the person's crown. Enter their body and witness the implant. Witness the tone being sent into the implant and destroying it, and then send the remains to God's light.

6. As soon as the process is finished, rinse yourself off and put yourself back into your space. Go into the Earth, pull Earth energy up through all your chakras to your crown chakra and make an energy break.

To permanently stop the person from having implants, use the belief work. Energy test for:

'I am impervious to attack.'
'I know how to live without being a victim.'

21

HEALING AND COMMUNICATING WITH ANIMALS

Some of the best friends that many of us have are our pets. They are the very essence of unconditional love. Some people become so attached to their pets that they are like children to them.

When you 'go in' to speak to an animal, you need to realize that most animals do not understand the spoken word. A much more realistic way to communicate with an animal is to form a picture and then telepathically transfer it to the animal's mind. Most animals don't intuitively send words, but use feelings, emotions and images.

It is also very important to understand that sending a feeling is very different from sending words. You are sending an emotion to the animal.

In the wild, animals can sense your fear, so it is important to send them feelings that they are safe and that you are safe. It is easy for them to accept intuitive love.

If you find yourself in a situation where you feel threatened by an animal, do not project the thought, 'Do not bite me.' Projecting any kind of image about biting may be misinterpreted, and you could cause a biting incident. Instead, if you find yourself in a situation with an aggressive animal, project pure love to the animal and move away slowly. Sending the projection of love telepathically will probably not work on all animals, however. Discretion is definitely the better part of valour when it comes to dealing with animals.

Someone once said that animals act upon pure instinct and it is only humans that have imagination. This person must not have studied animals. Animals have great imaginations and problem-solving abilities. They dream in much the same way as we do. Also, some animals, such as dogs and some cats, do understand words – not just a few occasional words, but whole sentences.

Animals can become chronically depressed, just like humans. If you have a dog that is depressed and lethargic, for example, you should project the picture of the animal in a happy situation with the master as its friend, giving it love.

It is easy to work on animals, even from long distances. They respond well to healing. But first, go up and ask their higher self for permission to do healing and belief work. Pull the disease from the animal and send it to the Creator of All That Is. Project the emotion or the feeling of the animal as strong and healthy.

Another way to work with animals is to go in and project to the animal that they are strong and healthy with a visualization.

Horses heal quickly, but they don't like to feel pain. It may be necessary to relieve their pain before witnessing the healing.

You may want to work on an animal's owner as well, as the animal often absorbs sickness from them. In the symbiotic relationship between the pet and master, the pet will attempt to heal their master by taking on emotions or the physical disease. Although animals are able to absorb sickness, they are often unable to get rid of it. This is why it is very important to clear your pet of negative energy on a regular basis. To do this, simply go up to the Seventh Plane and command that the energy be gone.

Animals usually respond quickly, but if they don't, they may need belief or feeling work.

Some of the feelings that animals may need are:

'I understand what it *feels like* to receive and accept love.'
'I know what it *feels like* to be loved.'
'I know what it *feels like* to be important.'
'I know how to live without feeling abandoned.'

22

AFFAIRS OF THE SOUL

For years I dreamed of a man that I was to be with later on in my life. I knew that he would have brown hair and blue eyes. As time passed, I knew that he would be from Montana. I knew that he would be a rancher or a farmer; I couldn't decide which one it would be, but I knew that it was one of the two, and I knew that he would have a child. When I first dreamed about him, I knew that he was married, but that he would be divorced. Later I knew that he would be driving an old blue and white truck and that his child was a young boy.

For some inexplicable reason I could not reach the man directly. It was through the dreams of the little boy that I attempted to reach him. I wanted the boy to tell his father that I was coming. For years I had intermittent dreams of becoming a great female wolf and running with a pack. In the form of this wolf I would run into the little boy's dreams and attempt to communicate that I was coming to see his father someday. I learned later that the recurring dreams terrified the little boy and he would wake up screaming and crying. These dreams went on for some years, with no success at communication.

In the meantime, I would always call the man 'my guy from Montana'. I asked the Creator time and time again what his name was, but I was told simply that he was 'my guy from Montana'.

I would tell my friends about the kind of man that I wanted, hoping that my man from Montana was 'the one'. I was having a discussion with one of my friends once, and I realize now that I was manifesting my soul mate, because I began to specify to her just what I needed in a man. I told her that I wanted one that was tall with blue eyes and brown hair. I told her that he had to be stable and I really wanted the man that I dreamed of, my man from Montana.

In 1997, I met a man whose name was Guy Stibal. (Get it? Stibal sounds like 'stable'.) When I saw my friend again she heard Guy's last name and said, 'Boy, can you manifest!' Guy was a farmer and a rancher. He farmed on the family farm in Idaho most of the year and he worked on the ranch in Montana in the summer. He told me that his son had dreamed for a long time about wolves that kept coming into his dreams and waking him up. I had seen this man in such detail that when I met him I thought the Creator was playing a joke on me, for certainly it couldn't be this easy.

To this day I know that the Creator gives you all the answers you need. My husband's name is Guy and he is from Montana: 'My Guy from Montana.' He is a partner with me on this journey, supporting me completely in the creation of ThetaHealing as we travel to different places in the world teaching people. This story is dedicated to him and I am also telling you it to remind you to trust your intuition.

SOUL MATES

Many people are confused by the phrase 'soul mate'. Most of this confusion is caused because there is more than one soul mate for each person on Earth. A soul mate is anyone that you have known from some other place in time – the pre-existence. Soul mates are sometimes compatible with you and sometimes not, but your heart will instinctively remember and love them. A soul mate has a magnetic pull that makes your heart beat faster and your palms become sweaty. They have something special inside. Your heart is excited to see them and when you are apart you can't wait to see them again.

I believe that since the year 1998 more soul mates have been finding each other than at any other time in history. Because of the change in the electromagnetic pull of the Earth and the spiritual development we are attaining, we are beginning to finally love ourselves. When you can truly love yourself, you're ready for a soul mate. Because a soul mate can make you happy or tear you apart, depending on how you feel about yourself. If you have not arrived at a point in time when you can truly love yourself, a soul-mate relationship will drag you over the coals.

As soon as you commence loving yourself, an interesting energy opens in the heart chakra. This energy triggers the sexual chakra, which calls to your soul mate. When you begin to call for your soul mate, you will find that you draw other people to you who are attracted to your energy. Not everyone that is going to be attracted to you is your soul mate. It is very important that you bring yourself the right mate to walk with you through life.

Be extremely careful when you ask for a soul mate; know exactly what you are asking for so that you will recognize that person when you find them. Also, when asking the Creator for a soul mate, make sure you ask for a *compatible* soul mate. Some people are confused and ask the Creator for a twin flame. A twin flame is someone who is exactly like you, and unless you truly like yourself, you will not find this match compatible.

Also remember that another person cannot make you complete; you must first be complete on your own. If you are not a whole person in and of yourself, then you have nothing to bring to a relationship.

Soul mates are part of the evolution of the Earth. Part of our evolution as human beings is to learn to accept others for who and what they are. It is very important that you do not romanticize so much about a partner that you don't see them for who they are. The term 'love is blind' applies to soul mates as well. It is imperative that when you find your soul mate, you accept them for who they are. As true partners, a couple can evolve and change together.

Many people are generous by nature and have a tendency to give all the time. Because of this they will draw soul mates to them that are not generous and take from the relationship more than they give. Be certain that you are ready for a soul mate to give you back the love that you give. Always make sure that you can accept and receive joy, and that you can accept and receive love. Energy test for the programme 'Love hurts' and replace it with the programme that the Creator tells you to replace it with.

The best way to find out if you are ready for a soul mate is with belief work.

Energy test for:

'I believe I can be loved by another person.'
'I can receive love from another person.'
'There is someone out there for me.'

These programmes should also be present in the other person for them to be your most compatible soul mate. In reading sessions I see women all the time who say, 'There is nothing out there but rotten men.' As a consequence, all they ever find are rotten men. I hear the same thing from the men that I talk to. They say, 'There is nothing out there but women who use men.' Because this is what they believe, this is all they find. Your subconscious will bring to you what it is told to.

There is a great deal of controversy around whether or not a person can love more than one person. After working with thousands of people, I have discovered that there is a gene for monogamy as well as a gene for non-monogamy, and I believe that a person can definitely love more than one person. But I also believe that the higher evolution of a being is to love one person totally and completely. I believe that to say that you love more than one person is a kind of cop-out, because then you're not obliged to know a person completely and to commit to them as a partner.

It is important to know that soul mates are out there and are very likely searching for you. It is possible to find the perfect soul mate for your life's journey.

THE PRINCIPLES OF SOUL MATES

- Soul families and soul mates are people whose spirits we recognize from other places and times. We seem to know them and can read their minds easily. Soul families have a tendency to travel through time together.
- There are more soul mates to choose from now than ever before. An individual has more than one compatible soul mate. One person may have dozens of soul mates, of many different ages, shapes and sizes.
- You must love yourself before calling in a soul mate. Once you manifest a soul mate, your level of development will dictate the soul mate that you draw from the Creative Force.
- People are drawn to one another for the negative that they have in common as well as the positive. You should remove as many negative beliefs as possible and do feeling work on yourself to draw to yourself the best person you can.
- A twin flame is someone exactly like you. They mirror you *exactly* and this may not be good.
- When you draw your soul mate to you through the Theta technique or another manifesting technique, be aware that you will attract other people to you as well, since your sexual chakra will be open. In the command process, it is important to state, 'I *have* my most compatible soul mate,' rather than saying, 'I *need* my most compatible soul mate.'
- You should specify that you receive the opposite or same sex, depending upon preference.
- Make a list of the criteria for the soul mate you wish to draw and state the complete list in your command.
- A compatible soul mate will flow with you. You will mesh with that individual with little or no friction. Usually you will have belief work to do together.
- Life is about choices. If you wish to leave your present relationship, this is between you and God. Ask God if your relationship could (or should) be saved and how, then decide to ask for a new soul mate.

- Do not ask for a *perfect* soul mate, since that person may be *too* perfect. Instead, ask for your *most compatible* soul mate.
- If you prefer someone to be faithful sexually, specify that they have a monogamy gene (which not everyone carries).

CALLING FOR YOUR MOST COMPATIBLE SOUL MATE

1. Centre yourself in your heart and visualize going down into Mother Earth, which is a part of All That Is.

2. Visualize bringing up energy through your feet, opening each chakra to the crown chakra. In a beautiful ball of light, go out to the universe.

3. Go beyond the universe, past the white lights, past the dark light, past the white light, past the jelly-like substance that is the Laws, into a pearly iridescent white light, into the Seventh Plane of Existence.

4. Make the command: *'Creator of All That Is, It is commanded that my most compatible soul mate be brought to me, and that they have these attributes: [state attributes]. Thank you! It is done. It is done. It is done.'*

5. Witness the call to your most compatible soul mate being sent out.

6. As soon as the process is finished, rinse yourself off and put yourself back into your space. Go into the Earth, pull Earth energy up through all your chakras to your crown chakra and make an energy break.

SOUL FRAGMENTS

As we have already seen, a soul fragment is a piece of essential life-force energy that is lost in intense emotional encounters. Soul fragments are exchanged through the history level. A soul fragment is more complex than a psychic hook. It is a fragment of another individual's life force that you have received or a fragment of your own that you have given to another individual. These exchanges may be either negative or positive and can be draining to the psyche.

Soul fragments may be lost or exchanged in the following ways:

- They may be lost with the death of a loved one with whom we have shared a lot.
- They may be lost in marriages or partnerships in which we have given a lot of ourselves. When you pull back your soul fragments from a past sexual partnership, you also bring back all the exchanges of DNA knowledge passed between both parties.

- When someone is ill, we can knowingly or unknowingly give something of ourselves over to them in an instinctual effort to heal them.
- Soul fragments may be lost in cases of rape or abuse.

Soul fragments may be the reason we still think of someone for years after leaving them and cannot make a healthy break from the memories. For example, if you continually think about an ex-husband, there may be a reason for it. You may still carry a soul fragment from that person. Please understand there's nothing wrong with thinking about them, but be sure that you are not continuing to give your power away to them and that you're not taking their power away from them.

To release and replace soul fragments from a particular person, make the command that all soul fragments that have been exchanged between you be rinsed clean and returned to both parties as follows:

THE SOUL FRAGMENT RETRIEVAL PROCESS

This exercise will do incredible things for your spiritual strength.

Two processes are given here. One is for another person; the other is for yourself.

1. Centre yourself in your heart and visualize going down into Mother Earth, which is a part of All That Is.

2. Visualize bringing up energy through your feet, opening each chakra to the crown chakra. In a beautiful ball of light, go out to the universe.

3. Go beyond the universe, past the white lights, past the dark light, past the white light, past the jelly-like substance that is the Laws, into a pearly iridescent white light, into the Seventh Plane of Existence.

4. Make the command:

   For someone else: 'Creator of All That Is, it is commanded that all soul fragments from all generations of time, eternity and between time from [person's name] be released, cleansed and returned to [state their name]. It is commanded that all soul fragments belonging to [person's name] be released, cleansed and returned to them. Thank you! It is done. It is done. It is done.'

   For yourself: 'Creator of All That Is, it is commanded that all soul fragments from all generations of time, eternity and between time from [person's name] be released from them, cleansed and returned to me, [name yourself]. It is *commanded that all soul fragments belonging to [person's name] be released from [name yourself], cleansed and returned to them as is proper for this time. Thank you! It is done. It is done. It is done.'*

5. Witness the fragments as they are returned.

6. As soon as the process is finished, rinse yourself off and put yourself back into your space. Go into the Earth, pull Earth energy up through all your chakras to your crown chakra and make an energy break.

ENERGETIC DIVORCE FROM PAST RELATIONSHIPS

One hidden programme that many people have is that of still believing that they are married to a person even when they are separated or physically divorced from them. If they became deeply attached to the other person, it may not matter if they were married or not, on an unconscious level they still believe that they are. Energy test them to find out if they still believe that they are married to the person energetically. The programme that will come up is 'I am married to [person's name]'. You would be surprised at how many people have not severed their energetic commitment to a past love.

THE PROCESS FOR ENERGETIC DIVORCE

1. Centre yourself in your heart and visualize going down into Mother Earth, which is a part of All That Is.

2. Visualize bringing up energy through your feet, opening each chakra to the crown chakra. In a beautiful ball of light, go out to the universe.

3. Go beyond the universe, past the white lights, past the dark light, past the white light, past the jelly-like substance that is the Laws, into a pearly iridescent white light, into the Seventh Plane of Existence.

4. Make the command: *'Creator of All That Is, it is commanded that [person's name] be released from the commitment of this marriage in the highest and best way. Thank you! It is done. It is done. It is done.'*

5. Witness the energy of the bond between the two people being sent to Creator's light.

6. As soon as the process is finished, rinse yourself off and put yourself back into your space. Go into the Earth, pull Earth energy up through all your chakras to your crown chakra and make an energy break.

23

MANIFESTING

Is your life what you make it? Or is it, as some say, all predestined and we have no choice but to simply exist without the ability to choose our destiny?

There are millions of people across the planet who follow the ideology that their life path is predestined and cannot be changed. These belief systems may be genetic, passed down from generation to generation. For those of us that refuse to follow the thread of fate that is spun without the consent of the soul, this ideology is impossible to accept. We accept that we are physical, but only in the sense that this is a small part of us. We insist that the majority of all that we are is spiritual in nature and is not dictated wholly by fate.

First let us be clear about our concept of reality. The mainstream idea is that it is the spiritual that is the illusion and the physical that is the reality. But what if we were to turn the tables on this concept to say it is the other way around, that the spiritual is the only real thing in existence and the physical is the illusion? What if we only think that we're here because our beliefs keep us here? If it is the physical that is the illusion then the reality of the spiritual can create changes in that illusion. If we could all see the infinite essence of the soul, the concept of manifesting in the physical world would not be so far-fetched.

In ThetaHealing, the concept of manifesting is the belief that it is possible to create something into the physical world using the power of the Creator of All That Is.

Every statement, thought and action is reflected by what we are manifesting in our lives. Every decision is made upon the mirror reflection of what we choose to create. What we think and say has a direct bearing upon whether our manifestations are for our benefit or detriment. If you constantly say that you are poor, you will be. If you constantly say and think that you are financially abundant, you will be. It is of the utmost importance to stay in a positive mind-set.

When deciding what it is you want to manifest in your life, the biggest challenge is deciding what it is that you truly want. Many people don't know what they want in their life, therefore they never create it. Other people believe that their life is leading them and they are not leading their life. These people go with the flow and wait to see what happens.

The truth is that we are creating our own reality and it is possible to manifest the best that the world has to offer. But you must first decide what it is you want in your life.

When I asked the Creator of All That Is to see truth I received more than I bargained for, as I've already told you. The most profound truth I was shown was that we have the ability to change our own reality. The Law of Truth showed me that it was possible to manifest through the Creator of All That Is. I was taken to the Seventh Plane of Existence where I could look down at the energy of my life. The Law said, 'Look! You can change anything! All you have to do is go up. Now look down at yourself, down at the energy of your life, and command change and it will be done.'

From that high lofty place that I came to know as the Seventh Plane of Existence, I reluctantly reached down into the energy of my life and manifested the changes I wanted. I witnessed the changes beginning to take shape and the Law was gone. I was back in my body to reflect upon the strange occurrences of the night. What was surprising to me was that over a short period of time all that I had manifested came to pass.

We all live in our own little world, our own version of reality. We are all busy doing our own thing, trying to fit in and be like everyone else. We think other people are like us, but they are not; similar perhaps, but not exactly like us. Everyone is unique. When you go up to the Seventh Plane of Existence, you can view yourself and your world and see what is going on in your life. From this perspective you can command changes for the highest and best (see below).

SPONTANEOUS MANIFESTATIONS

After the Law of Truth had showed me how to manifest, I began to have spontaneous manifestations. The more readings I did, the more often I was in a deep Theta state. Even when I was not doing readings I was in a mild state of Theta wave and it seemed that much of what I said and thought would come to pass in the near future. These spontaneous manifestations began to occur closer to the time that I thought of them, sometimes immediately after they were spoken about. They began when I mentioned the things I desired during readings.

THE TOPAZ RING

I did a reading on a woman and asked her where she had got the beautiful amethyst ring that she was wearing. I mentioned that I would love to have a blue topaz ring. I was undoubtedly in a Theta state when I made this statement. I remember thinking that it was a really beautiful ring and I just left it at that. Two days later I received a gift from a separate source in the form of a blue topaz ring!

THE AMETHYST GEODE

Not long after the ring incident, I was talking to a friend and mentioned that I wanted a large amethyst geode to put in the corner of my healing room. I told her that I wanted it to be about 2 feet high. A couple of days later a gentleman came into my office and told me that he had something that belonged to me. It was an amethyst geode. He needed someone to come with him to help him pick it up and deliver it. He said that he couldn't lift it alone because it weighed 230 pounds and was about 2 feet high and 2½ feet across.

After this, the manifestations began to increase in intensity. Containers of fluid filled themselves up and the things that I thought and talked about began to come into my life. My gas tank even filled itself up and a large dent in my car went back to normal. These occurrences were witnessed by others.

The Law of Truth that came into my living room so many years ago still comes to visit me at least two or three times a year to see what I've manifested in my life and to give me further guidance. What the Law comes to remind me is that you can manifest anything. It showed me that the way that we perceive the world is an illusion and that we only think that we're here. Our DNA just needs to be reprogrammed so that we can create and re-create our existence with light in multiples of cells every 16-billionth of a second.

THE DIFFERENT FORMS OF MANIFESTING

Just talking about things will sometimes manifest them in your life; the chances of this happening are about 30 to 40 per cent. Visualizing increases your chances to nearer 50 per cent. But a Theta state increases the likelihood enormously. Being in a Theta state while manifesting will increase the chances of manifestation to about 80 to 90 per cent.

THE PRINCIPLES OF MANIFESTING

You are only allowed to manifest for *your* life. You are not allowed to manifest for others. For instance, you cannot manifest a job for your spouse. Neither can you can make someone love you. No matter how much you want them to, this is down to their free will.

You could also use this technique to manifest new guides in your life. However, when doing this, always ask for a guide that is more intelligent than you are but not so intelligent that you can't understand what they say.

One important thing to remember when you are doing any kind of manifesting is that you will get exactly what you ask for. Always ask for the highest and the best. If you need money, be mindful that you ask for it in the *highest and the best way*. For example, you do not want to get a lot of money from an accident insurance claim filed on behalf of yourself.

To sum up:

- We create our own reality.
- You cannot manifest the love of a specific someone.
- You are only allowed to manifest in your own life.
- You may use manifesting to bring in new spirit guides.
- Be specific as to what you ask for. If you ask for a lot of money, specify that it comes to you in the highest and best way.
- Know exactly what you want, 'word for word', and specify 'word for word' in your prayer of manifestation.
- Be careful with the spoken word and directed thought forms, as this may bring manifestations, either good or bad, to your life. What you say and what you think creates your life.
- State the manifestation in the present positive sense: 'I have this now!'
- Don't command that you change to be like someone else; rather command that you be the best that *you* can be.

There are two manifesting techniques that have proven themselves to me time and time again. The first is the one that I was shown by the Law of Truth and the other is the Kahuna *Manna* Manifestation from Hawaii.

MANIFESTING WITH THE SEVENTH PLANE OF EXISTENCE

If you want to create something for yourself, proceed as follows:

THE PROCESS OF MANIFESTING FROM THE SEVENTH PLANE OF EXISTENCE

1. Begin by sending your consciousness down into the centre of Mother Earth, which is a part of All That Is.
2. Visualize bringing up energy through your feet, opening each chakra to the crown chakra. In a beautiful ball of light, go out to the universe.
3. Go beyond the universe, past the white lights, past the dark light, past the white light, past the jelly-like substance that is the Laws, into a pearly iridescent white light, into the Seventh Plane of Existence.
4. Look into your life and see what is going on; see the things that need to be changed.
5. See your life like a bubble of energy, and yourself as a giant whose arm reaches from the Seventh Plane into the bubble. Reach into it with your mental arm and imagine stirring it to create the changes.
6. As you do this, command the changes you desire.
7. Feel the essence of what you have just commanded; experience it as though it is already done.
8. As soon as the process is finished, rinse yourself off and put yourself back into your space. Go into the Earth, pull Earth energy up through all your chakras to your crown chakra and make an energy break.

Just be careful what you ask for, you just might get it!

KAHUNA *MANNA* MANIFESTATION

The ancient Hawaiians believed that there was an essential force, called *manna*, that pervaded all things. It could be breathed into the body to create manifestations and bring about healing. The Hawaiian Kahunas believe that the higher self manifests the physical self and that something is not made of nothing. So they gather the *manna* energy, the life force around them, and send it up to the higher self to create the manifestation.

THE PROCESS FOR KAHUNA *MANNA* MANIFESTATION

Prior to beginning, have in mind the object or situation you have chosen to manifest in your life.

1. To begin, sit down with your legs uncrossed and become very relaxed.

2. Expel all the air from your lungs. Do this by exhaling the air from the lungs, then literally forcing out more air by using short exhaling puffs. This removes all of the old air from the lungs, making room for a large amount of *manna*.

3. Take a deep breath, taking it in all the way and pushing the air deep into the belly, ballooning the belly, and hold for 30 seconds. If you are a woman, this is all you do before you release the breath. If you are a man, you take another breath in (before exhaling the belly breath) to fill up the chest. (With *manna* energy, the life force is held in the stomach for the woman and the chest for the man.)

4. Hold the breath for 30 seconds and then release.

5. Take in another deep breath and push the air deep into the belly (men need to take another inhalation, same as before), hold for 30 seconds and release. As you hold the air, you imagine the *manna*, the life-force energy, going through your body and nourishing every cell as light.

6. As you release the air the second time, you take a third deep breath in, doing exactly the same as before (with men taking another inhalation to fill up the chest), holding for 30 seconds and releasing.

7. On the fourth breath, place your hands out in front of you as though you were holding a ball. Imagine a ball of energy being built up between your hands as you take the next deep breath in and push it down into the belly. (If you are a man, take another inhalation to fill up the chest.) Hold for 30 seconds and release.

8. As you take in the next deep breath, feel the energy building, becoming stronger and stronger. Imagine the ball of light growing. Push the air into the belly (with an extra inhalation for the men to fill up the chest), hold for 30 seconds and release.

9. On the sixth and final breath, take a deep breath in, push the air into the belly (men, take an extra inhalation to fill up chest) and hold for 30 seconds. As you near completion of holding the breath, imagine the ball of energy going into your solar plexus, up through your heart, up through your throat, up through your crown chakra and about six feet above your head.

10. At this time you command the energy by saying, '*I have this in my life now. Thank you! It is done. It is done. It is done.*' This command can be made while holding the breath or when you exhale – both are acceptable.

11. It is very important to send a picture to your subconscious of exactly what you have chosen to manifest. Sending a picture to your higher self tells it what you want in your life. Command it to be so and so it is, now.

12. When you have finished, rinse yourself off and put yourself back into your space.

This Hawaiian Kahuna technique is especially efficient and has many magnificent qualities.

Finally, be aware that there be may be blocks on some levels concerning what you want to manifest. If your manifestations do not come into reality, the cause may be programmes on core, genetic, history or soul levels. Test for these programmes and replace accordingly.

24

THE FUTURE READING

Do you remember the Y2K scare in the year 1999? It was said that all the computers in the world were going to crash in 2000. So many people thought that there was going to be chaos, confusion, mass anarchy and electrical failures, not to mention rioting in the streets. This was all because computers might not recognize a number.

All of my clients asked me about the outcome of this supposed looming disaster. When I went up and asked about Y2K, God said that all would be fine. I asked a specific question and I received the specific answer, 'No, this will not happen and it will be OK, but there will be a great sale on generators directly after.' Accepting this answer was a step of faith for me, because group consciousness had created a hysteria that said, 'We are all doomed!' My friend Kevin was certain that Y2K was going to happen. Even a client that was the wife of a general in the army told me to watch out and stay indoors. But I trusted in the message and told everyone that I knew that all would be fine. I even planned a pot luck dinner for New Year's Eve, inviting all of my metaphysical friends. They nearly all called me, graciously bowing out, fearful of leaving their homes. Only four came. The majority were afraid that something would happen when the clock struck 12.

Midnight came and went without mishap, and so did Y2K, just as God said it would. This shows you that we should not let our fears rule us, our computers control us or group consciousness interfere with truth in a future reading.

Only the journey is written, not the destination. The future is not set in stone; it constantly changes with the choices we make.

The truth about future reading is that a person is creating their own future with their thoughts, deeds and actions. The practitioner can only tell them what they are creating at that moment. They can alter what the practitioner has seen by changing their lifestyles and patterns. For instance, if a person is on the verge of losing a job, they can always change the energy that is causing this to happen and keep their job. Similarly, if you see a divorce in your client's future, advising them of it gives them the opportunity to prevent it from becoming a reality.

It is important for you to explain this to your clients. What you see is the path they are walking at that time. But life has infinite possibilities and the future is always changeable. Any time that you give a client advice and they change their lifestyle and patterns because of it, the original future has been changed to a new one.

A future reading is a very important, very powerful thing. You must be extremely careful not to mislead your clients by making decisions for them. You cannot tell them what choices to make or how to live their life. That is not your responsibility, it is theirs. You cannot tell them to leave someone who is hurting them, you can only tell them what you see as their possible or most likely future. All decisions concerning what they are going to do about a situation must be made by them. Each one of us is weaving a pattern, a mosaic that represents our life.

FAITH IN THE ANSWER

When doing a future reading it is very important to know that your questions will be answered specifically by the Creator. For instance, I had a woman who kept asking me where her next mate was coming from, and every time I did a future reading for her, I kept getting over and over again that the man she was looking for would ask her for coffee three times. His father would be in a wheelchair and she would be a caregiver for the father and the man that she was looking for was right behind her. She waited very impatiently for this man to arrive.

She worked for a hospice and one of her assignments was to take care of a man in a wheelchair. While doing this, she met his son. During his visits to see his father, he asked her for coffee three times. He also asked her several times for her phone number and, at last, reluctantly, she obliged. Then he lost her phone number, so looked her name up in the phone book. She was astonished when he called her to say, 'Oh my gosh! You will never believe this, but you live right behind me. In fact, your bedroom window is facing my back yard.'

When I had asked where the man was, the Creator had answered, 'Right behind her.' I had asked an exact question and in return I had received an exact answer. At the time it had made no sense to anyone, but it could not have been more accurate.

The more you use this technique, the better you will become at wording your questions. With experience, you will improve at asking specific questions and interpreting the answers. And you must remember that to make ThetaHealing work for you, you must keep your opinions to yourself, which is a challenge all its own.

THE PRINCIPLES OF FUTURE READING

At some point in time you will find yourself faced with a client who has questions pertaining to the future. This is no challenge since there is always the connection with the Creator, and it is the Creator that does the reading. However, there are a few guidelines to go by.

Explain to the client that the future is not set and that there are many possible futures for any one person. The future changes with our choices and with the choices of other people. We all have free will to create a good future, or perhaps create a difficult one. When you do a future reading on a client, you are giving the person the most likely scenario based on the particular choice the person makes.

Example question: 'Will I be fired from my job?' Answer: 'Yes, if you don't do your job, you will. If you want to keep your job, you must apply yourself.'

THE FUTURE READING PROCESS

1. Centre yourself in your heart and visualize going down into Mother Earth, which is a part of All That Is.

2. Visualize bringing up energy through your feet, opening each chakra to the crown chakra. In a beautiful ball of light, go out to the universe.

3. Go beyond the universe, past the white lights, past the dark light, past the white light, past the jelly-like substance that is the Laws, into a pearly iridescent white light, into the Seventh Plane of Existence.

4. Make the command: *'Creator of All That Is, grant me a future reading on [name the person]. Thank you! It is done. It is done. It is done.'*

5. Go through their crown chakra into the body. Pull your consciousness up and hold your vision on the left side of their body (your right side).

6. Have the client ask questions that pertain to their life. You will see flashes of scenarios that are going on in their life from the past, present and future. Ask the Creator to specify which is past, present and future, and you will be shown. You will be given an actual account of what is going on.

7. As soon as the process is finished, rinse yourself off and put yourself back into your space. Go into the Earth, pull Earth energy up through all your chakras to your crown chakra and make an energy break.

Θ *The future of a client will automatically change when they have belief programmes removed and replaced. It is a good idea to do a future reading after any belief work has been done in a session.*

25

DNA

I have included this explanation of DNA to help you to understand the mechanics and mystery that is inside each living being on this planet. Some years ago the concept of energy healing at a DNA level was shown to me in the DNA activation and the gene replacement processes (*see the following two chapters*). Both of these techniques employ ThetaHealing to heal on a submicroscopic level, in a world so infinitely tiny that it is a universe all of its own.

DNA (deoxyribonucleic acid) can be perceived as a library containing all the genetic information that a cell needs to sustain and reproduce itself. It is, in effect, the blueprint for the functions of the cell. In order to accomplish these functions, DNA must contain a detailed blueprint for synthesizing the enzymes required to perform every activity of the cell. If any part of this blueprint is missing or inaccurate, the cell will not function properly and could even die. So DNA may be thought of as the blueprint for life.

DNA is found in the nuclei and mitochondria of tissue cells. It is found in two forms in the nucleus: as chromatin or as chromosomes. Chromatin is made of uncoiled DNA strands wrapped around histone protein cores. It resembles a string with beads. The bead structure is called a nucleosome. When a cell begins the reproductive process, the chromatin becomes more tightly coiled and is transformed into tiny rod-shaped chromosomes.

DNA is composed of two long chains of nucleic acid molecules twisted around one another in the form of a double helix. These strands are made up of building blocks called nucleotides, consisting of a phosphate group, a five-carbon deoxyribose sugar and an organic base. The organic base of a DNA strand can be one of four kinds: G-guanine, C-cytosine, A-adenine or T-thymine. Because of their special molecular shapes and electrical patterns, guanine will bond only with cytosine, and adenine will bond only with thymine. The deoxyribose and phosphate group are joined to form the backbone of the chain of molecules. Attached to the deoxyribose sugar of this DNA backbone are the organic bases. These organic bases are bound by weak hydrogen bonds to the bases of the second chain of DNA molecules.

A set of three consecutive nucleotides in a strand of DNA is called a triplet or a codon. Each triplet contains the code for one of the 20 amino acids, the building blocks that form proteins. Sometimes several combinations of triplets are required to design an amino acid. The sequence in each segment of DNA determines which protein is synthesized.

DNA contains the genetic codes that instruct chemical compounds in the synthesis of proteins that control specific cell functions. A gene is a segment of a DNA molecule. The nucleotide sequence of each segment contains the genetic information for making one kind of protein molecule. Genes tell a cell how to synthesize protein molecules that function as structural materials, enzymes and other vital substances. Therefore, genes determine a person's gender, eye colour and skin colour, hair colour, blood type and so forth.

Chromosomes are located in the nucleus of a cell. A chromosome is made up of DNA molecules coiled around a protein framework. The number of chromosomes within the cells of an organism varies from species to species. For example a domestic cat's cells have 38 chromosomes, a dog's cells have 78 and a human's cells have 46.

The human genome is the set of genetic information encoded in the 46 chromosomes found in the nucleus of each cell. The chromosomes are organized in 23 pairs; one chromosome of each pair is inherited from the father and one from the mother.

Thus the human genome is comprised of very long DNA molecules corresponding to each chromosome. Arranged along these DNA molecules are the genes. The quest of the human genome project is to determine the nucleotide sequence, the location and the identity of each of the human genes. The task has relied on automated machines that sequence the DNA and computer programmes that search for and identify genes. A rough draft of the human genome was completed in the summer of 2000.

If you were to uncoil the DNA from a cell, it would stretch out to be two yards long and ten atoms wide. This thread is a billon times longer that its width. It is 120 times narrower than the smallest wavelength of visible light and cannot be seen with regular microscopes. This two-yard long thread is coiled into a cell whose nucleus is in volume two millionths of a pinhead. A human has an estimated 100 thousand billion cells, with the possibility of 125 billion miles of DNA in the body. This length would wrap around the Earth five million times!

Scientists do not understand at least a third of the DNA in the human genome and in the past they termed it 'junk DNA'. What this means to the rest of us is that this extra DNA is an unknown, an enigma if you will.

In the early 1980s, scientists developed a sophisticated measuring device to demonstrate that the cells of living beings emit photons. They found that the cells emit photons up to 100 units per second, per square centimetre (half an inch) of surface area. They also showed that the DNA was the source of this photon emission. This means that the DNA is emitting a quantum of *visible light*.

By volume, DNA contains over a trillion times more information capability than our most sophisticated storage devices. It is biological technology of the highest order.

DNA and its mechanisms are the same for all creatures great and small. The only thing that changes from species to species is the order of the letters (sugars). It is thought that DNA has remained constant for at least three billion years. For instance, 400 human genes match similar genes in yeast. This means that all life on this planet has the same building blocks, from the smallest bacteria to an eight-ton elephant.

Francis Crick, who co-discovered DNA, wrote a book entitled *Life Itself: Its Origin and Nature*. In this book, Crick states that the DNA molecule is unable to build itself on its own. Proteins are needed for this, but proteins alone are incapable of reproducing themselves without the blueprint of the DNA. For there to be life there must be a synthesis of these two molecular systems. Crick estimates that the chances that the emergence of one single protein that would build the first DNA is not likely, even remote. Further, the complex chain of events leading up to what we know today as DNA could not have happened by chance. Crick suggests that DNA is *cosmic* in origin.

Science has found that there are genetic sequences known as 'master genes' that control hundreds of other genes like an on–off switch. These master genes send messages to create, for instance, the intricate structures of the human eye.

In ThetaHealing, DNA is the microcosm to healing the macrocosm of the human body. *Healing* is clarified by not only making the body well, but also healing the mind and the spirit. This is done by changing the messages that are sent to the DNA.

26

THE DNA ACTIVATION TECHNIQUE

DNA activation is a gift from the Creator as an opening to our intuitive gifts. It allows us to survive the environmental poisons created by humankind, as well as accelerate our psychic senses. As a species we are now evolving and are waking up dormant parts of our spiritual DNA. The DNA activation is becoming a part of the Earth's collective consciousness. Enough people have been activated for it to happen spontaneously, without the aid of a practitioner. Many people have already intuitively activated themselves.

TURNING THE DREAM INTO REALITY

I was told by the Creator that when enough people have been activated, the whole of the Earth's consciousness will move up in its vibration. When this happens, people will automatically be activated from the collective consciousness that we all share. I believe that this activation will happen automatically in the future in 12 to 24 years. With the activation and other techniques in this book, we have been given an opportunity by the Creator to use our intuitive abilities in the next phase of our evolution. This evolution is the next level of human consciousness.

In the activation, we are activating strands to the DNA and its existing 46 chromosomes in what will be explained as the master cell of the brain. The mitochondrial DNA is also activated.

From the moment that the activation was performed upon me, my life began to change. I can remember being on my massage table witnessing the activation in my head. When it was finished I got up and I knew that I was changed forever. My first thought was that I would get a divorce. (The activation is not a license for divorce!) It was after that that I found my soul mate, Guy. In the days and weeks that followed I had strange metaphysical experiences. When I was doing massages and readings my hands would disappear. I witnessed containers in my refrigerator refill themselves. I saw rubbing alcohol refill itself in the seconds between my putting it down and picking it up. Most of the people who have had DNA activation have had similar experiences.

THE PINEAL GLAND

Located in the middle of the brain is a small gland called the *pineal gland*. This gland has been called the 'house of the soul' and it has been referred to as such for thousands of years.

Initially, modern science believed that the pineal gland was a completely non-functional gland or that its functions were not understood. It was thought that the *pituitary* gland controlled everything in the body. The scientific world has changed its view since discovering that the pineal gland releases many substances that direct the pituitary in its function. It was only after the 1960s that scientists discovered that the pineal gland was responsible for the production of melatonin, which is regulated in a circadian rhythm (the body's time clock). Melatonin is a derivative of the amino acid tryptophan, which also has other functions in the central nervous system. The production of melatonin by the pineal gland is stimulated by darkness and inhibited by light.

You don't have to be a scientist to do the DNA activation technique, but you should know that the pineal gland is located exactly in the centre of the brain, directly down from the crown and at the back of the third eye.

THE MASTER CELL

Within the pineal gland is what is called the *master cell*, and it is this cell that is the operation centre for all the other cells in the body. The master cell is the starting point of healing for many of the functions that the body performs. Within it is the chromosome of DNA that is the heart of the DNA activation.

Inside the master cell is a tiny universe all its own that is a master key to our function. It runs everything in the body, from the colour of our hair to the way we wiggle our feet. All parts of the body are controlled by the programmes in the chromosomes and the DNA. And inside the master cell are the youth and vitality chromosomes.

THE YOUTH AND VITALITY CHROMOSOMES

You have 46 chromosomes (23 pairs of two strands each) in your body and each of those chromosomes has two strands of DNA. The first two that you are going to be working on within the master cell are called the youth and vitality chromosomes. These chromosomes are always in pairs, so if you activate one you obviously have to work on the other.

I believe that the youth and vitality chromosomes are called the chronos and maintain track of the seconds, minutes and hours of the day for the body. They contain memory materials that are called *shadow strands*.

THE SHADOW STRANDS

When you are inside the master cell you will witness the Creator beginning to build parts of the ladder to bring into physical form the shadow strands. These are the invisible memories of the youth and vitality chromosome, waiting to be formed and awakened to bring us back to the Creator of All That Is. In the evolution of humankind the accumulation of negative memories and feelings changed part of the chromosomes and DNA. This lowered our resistance to different diseases. Only a memory remained of these changes in the form of the shadow strands.

In the DNA activation you will witness the shadow strands forming new parts to the chromosomal ladder. These new parts of the ladder are formed from amino acids (sugars) that build new strands from the memory of the old. You will watch as they build one by one until they have climbed up eight rungs of the ladder. Each side is counted as one step, so there is a total of 16 steps. After this climbing and building process you will see strands of *rainbow light* come into the chromosome and be capped off at the top with a beautiful pearl iridescent white cap that looks like a shoestring top. This is called the *telomere*; it is responsible for our staying young.

THE TELOMERE

Telomeres are composed of repeating sequences and various proteins, and act to protect the terminal ends of chromosomes. This prevents chromosomal fraying and keeps the ends of the chromosomes from being processed as a double-strand DNA break. Telomeres are extended by telomerases, specialized reverse enzymes that are involved in synthesis of telomeres in humans and many other, but not all, organisms.

As we get older, telomeres become thinner and worn. If they become too short, they will potentially unfold from their closed structure. It is thought that the cell detects this uncapping as DNA damage and then will enter cellular ageing, growth arrest or apoptosis, depending on the cell's genetic background. Apoptosis is a form of cell death necessary to make way for new cells and to remove cells whose DNA has been damaged to the point at which cancerous change is liable to occur. Uncapped telomeres also result in chromosomal fusions. Since this damage cannot be repaired in normal somatic cells, the cell may even go into apoptosis. Many age-related diseases are linked to shortened telomeres. Organs deteriorate as more and more of their cells die off or enter cellular ageing. This is why it is so important that you witness the telomere being formed on the end of the chromosome.

THE LAWS OF TIME

When the command is made that the activation be done, the Creator shows you the process in a version that your mind can accept. The second you are into the master cell you are bending the Laws of Time. The work that you are doing takes place in a fraction of a second, so for you to actually see it, your brain has to slow it down to visualize it. All you have to say to visualize it is 'Creator, show me.'

THE ACTIVATION PROCESS

This is the process that I was given:

PART ONE: ACTIVATION OF THE YOUTH AND VITALITY CHROMOSOMES COMMAND PROCESS

1. Ground and centre yourself in your heart and visualize going down into Mother Earth, which is a part of All That Is.

2. Visualize bringing up energy through your feet, opening up all of your chakras as you go. Go up out of your crown, out to the universe.

3. Go beyond the universe, past the white lights, past the dark light, past the white light, past the jelly-like substance that is the Laws, into a pearly iridescent white light, into the Seventh Plane of Existence.

4. In silence, make the command: *'Creator of All That Is, it is commanded that the activation of the youth and vitality chromosomes of [client's name] take place on this day. Thank you! It is done. It is done. It is done. Show me the master cell in the pineal gland.'*

5. Observe the virtual DNA strands stack in pairs on top of each other with a telomere cap at the ends. Sometimes this happens so fast that you may have to ask the Creator for a replay later.

6. As soon as you see that the process is finished, rinse yourself off and put yourself back into your space. Go into the Earth, pull Earth energy up through all your chakras to your crown chakra and make an energy break.

Part one of the DNA activation is now complete.

Since in this first procedure you are making cellular changes in the body from the master cell, the body will begin to purge toxins. Some people may experience a healing cleanse, a period of detoxification and purification. Others might experience toxins coming out of their system on all levels – spiritually, mentally, emotionally and physically.

Generally, there should be a space of time between the two activations. Some people, however, are ready for both of them simultaneously. With these people you may do the second step immediately after the first if they are ready to receive it. The way that you can tell if they can immediately receive the second part of the activation is to stay in their space as the first part is finishing. As you are in their pineal gland, you will witness the remaining chromosomes beginning to come to life on their own. If you see this, the person is ready for the second activation. You will witness the addition of 10 new strands to the remaining 44.

MITOCHONDRIA

In the second process you will be activating mitochondria as well, which accelerates the process. In cell biology, a mitochondrion (plural mitochondria) is an organelle, variants of which are found in most eukaryotic cells. Mitochondria possess their own genetic material and the machinery to manufacture their own RNAs and proteins. The 46 chromosomes in the cell nucleus is the blueprint, but the mitrochondria hold the energy, the ATP that makes it all function. Mitochondria are sometimes described as 'cellular power plants', because their primary function is to convert organic materials into energy in the form of ATP.

Usually a cell has hundreds or thousands of mitochondria, which can occupy up to 25 per cent of the cell's cytoplasm. Mitochondria have their own DNA and are accepted by endosymbiotic theory to have descended from once free-living bacteria.

PART TWO: ACTIVATION OF THE REMAINING CHROMOSOMES

The next step in the process is as follows:

1. Centre yourself in your heart and visualize going down into Mother Earth, which is a part of All That Is.

2. Visualize bringing up energy through your feet, opening each chakra to the crown chakra. In a beautiful ball of light, go out to the universe.

3. Go beyond the universe, past the white lights, past the dark light, past the white light, past the jelly-like substance that is the Laws, into a pearly iridescent white light, into the Seventh Plane of Existence.

4. In silence, make the command: *'Creator of All That Is, it is commanded that the remaining chromosomes be activated.* [This awakens the mitrochondria.] *Thank you! It is done. It is done. It is done. Show me the master cell in the pineal gland.'*

5. As soon as you envision the process as finished, rinse yourself off and imagine your energy coming back into your space. Go into the Earth, pull Earth energy up through all of your chakras to the crown chakra and make an energy break.

AFTER-EFFECTS

Depending on the health of the individual, there may be a period of detoxification after the DNA activation. Most people experience a slight cleansing with cold-like symptoms and some people ache all over. I suggest as a remedy that they take a little calcium and perhaps a little chelated zinc.

WORDS BECOME REALITY

The one thing I have found to be consistent with the activation is that the likelihood of the spoken word and strong thoughts becoming reality increases dramatically after it is done. So, once the activation begins to take effect, it is important to stay positive and affirm that you have abundance coming into your life. Do not affirm lack in your life, because after the activation your words and thoughts will be 10 times more powerful and must be focused in the right direction.

When you're working with the energetic DNA, the negative aspects of your life will begin to be replaced with positive aspects.

THE COMPANY THAT YOU KEEP

DNA activation brings us to a higher spiritual vibration. Our family and friends may not be on the same vibrational level and the activation increases our awareness of the negative influences of others. So, if you have an associate or friend that is not for your highest and best good you will easily and gently gravitate away from them. If you are in an unhappy relationship, you either will remove yourself from that relationship or make it better.

Once the activation has been done within yourself, it should also be done on your spouse, because your dual spiritual vibration needs to accelerate together or you may choose to be apart. It is possible that the activation will happen by sleeping with your spouse. This is because cell talks to cell, but you must be patient, as this will take several months.

AWAKENED MASTERS

The DNA activation is a part of the awakening of the masters on Earth. This is the story of how I was told to teach the masters this work.

Over the years I have been given many gifts by the energy of the Hawaiian islands. One of these came in the form of a busted seminar. One of my first teachers moved to Honolulu and set up a class for me with a woman that he had been working with named Teresa. She was an osteopath with a life-long interest in metaphysics and spirituality. This was to be my first trip to the island of Oahu. Then a mild disaster struck. Two weeks before the seminar, I received a call from Teresa. It seems that the teacher had had some misunderstandings with her and skipped out on the seminar, leaving Teresa and her partner, Larry, to hold the bag. Teresa told me all that had happened and asked if I would come in spite of the situation.

I knew that it was likely to be a small class, but God told me that there was a good reason to go. I was told that more would come from the trip, and in the end, it did.

Because the seminar had become disorganized, it was a small class of seven people. Most of these were wonderful; however, there were a few who were difficult. One of the women was a hateful person who attempted to attack me at every opportunity. She even attempted to demean my husband. She was the kind of person who elevates themselves at the expense of others. I was tempted simply to leave and go home, but something told me to finish the class, difficult as it was. Needless to say, I was a little discouraged by the conduct of some of the class members.

When the class was over, I went to Hana, Maui, to visit some friends. We stayed as their guests and it was a beautiful house with commanding views of the flora and fauna that are typical of Hana. Night came and with it the magical timelessness that is peculiar to Hawaii. The trade winds billowed the curtains all night, and continued to do so even when we closed the glass doors tight. Guy and I had strange dreams all night.

Morning came and I was in the bathroom when a voice came to me that seemed to speak all around me. It was one that I've known forever. It was Pele, the goddess of Hawaii. She said to me, 'Vianna, you know that you should only teach the *masters* this work. You told the Creator that you'd teach anyone who needed this work. But teach only the masters who appreciate and respect this work. Just because people need it doesn't mean they understand or appreciate it. Change your intention.' I realized then that I was asking for the people who needed the work instead of the people who were ready for the work. This visitation made me feel better about life.

Later that day, my friend Lani came down from her mountain to see me. She very rarely leaves her mountain. She is a wonderful healer and she looked like a goddess as she walked up to me and said, 'Vianna, I have a message for you from the goddess Pele: only teach the masters that appreciate and respect this work.'

This was pure validation for me – receiving the message physically as well as spiritually. From that time on I asked the Creator to send only the masters that appreciated and accepted this work. My students changed immediately and became less driven by the ego and more by divinity. Since then the teachers and students who have come to learn ThetaHealing have, for the most part, been ascended masters in human form that love and cherish the work.

This is why ThetaHealing is so easy for the people who come to learn it – many are awakened masters who have been assigned to develop the goodness in humankind. They have come back to Earth to make sure that we are ready to graduate to goodness. As already mentioned, it is easier for a master to be born as a human on this plane rather than lower their vibration from another plane. This way, their energy is in a marriage with this place and time. The master is then able to complete their mission here. It is easier to raise vibrational energy than it is to lower it.

27

GENE REPLACEMENT

The reason that I have the gene work near the end of this book is not because it is difficult to perform. Once you understand it, it is easy. However, it is imperative that you understand the reading, the healing and the belief work before doing gene replacement. Belief work can influence the genes; in and of itself it will *indirectly* repair damage to the physical DNA. The gene replacement process is a guide to *directly* changing a physical genetic defect in the DNA. It is actually the easiest thing to do in ThetaHealing.

Physical DNA is composed of hydrogen bonds. In chemistry, a hydrogen bond is the easiest bond to change. This means that thoughts focused in the correct way can affect DNA.

When you change a physical gene, the process occurs so quickly that you may not be aware that it has been done. All that you are likely to see is a flash of light. The actual changing of the gene takes only a fraction of a second. The key to ThetaHealing is to witness the healing, so ask for a slow-motion replay if you choose to see more. However, *the flash is the witness that brings it into reality*.

THE PRINCIPLES OF GENE REPLACEMENT

1. To change or restructure any physical genetic code, you must have verbal permission from the person.
2. Inside the DNA are recordings that make the systems of the body function. These recordings affect memories, feelings and defects, which, in turn, affect particular body parts that are making the system work. Genetic defects are held in some of these recordings.
3. Visualize the recordings inside the pineal gland in the master cell. This is where the changes are made.

4. In the master cell of the pineal gland, visualize the pillar of DNA. Make the command to be taken to the area of the DNA portion that is to be changed.
5. Visualize the affected or defective portion of the DNA being pulled. In addition, watch the four-square (four-part) cubicle shown to you with the parts:

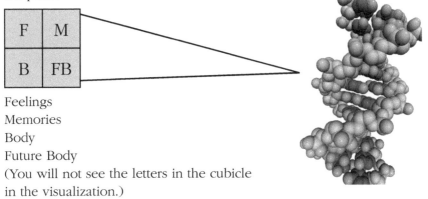

F	M
B	FB

Feelings
Memories
Body
Future Body
(You will not see the letters in the cubicle in the visualization.)

The changes made in the master cell will be replicated throughout the entire body.

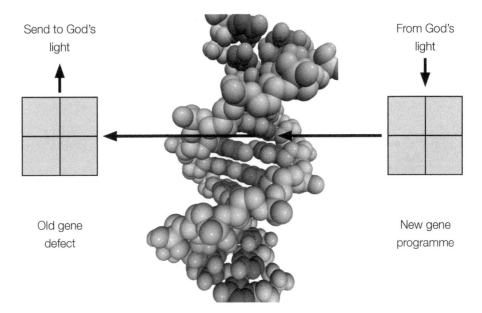

Send to God's light — Old gene defect

From God's light — New gene programme

In respect of medical conditions, all that you need to do is watch the Creator rearranging the DNA genes/nucleic structure. Since all medical defects come in pairs, both genes of the pair need to be changed. To make the gene/nucleic changes, command that the correct rearrangement be made and observe the Creator making it.

Be aware that the results from gene work may take a little time, since the new codes will not be in effect until the new cells have replaced the old cells in the defective area.

Environmental conditions may cause difficulties in the DNA encoding and may change the structure of the DNA over time. To work on a dysfunctional gene clip, follow this process:

THE GENE REPLACEMENT PROCESS

Ask for verbal permission and then do the following:

1. Centre yourself in your heart and visualize going down into Mother Earth, which is a part of All That Is.

2. Visualize bringing up energy through your feet, opening each chakra to the crown chakra. In a beautiful ball of light, go out to the universe.

3. Go beyond the universe, past the white lights, past the dark light, past the white light, past the jelly-like substance that is the Laws, into a pearly iridescent white light, into the Seventh Plane of Existence.

4. Make the command: *'Creator of All That Is, it is commanded to heal this gene in [person's name] to change it in the highest and best way. Show me.'*

5. Now go into the person's space.

6. First, ask the Creator to show you the defective gene. Then go to the master cell in the pineal.

If you see this,

a visualization of a DNA helix, then it is a matter of rearranging nucleic acid. This tells us that it is a physical defect caused by a pollutant in the mother or father's genetic code. The factors that may have caused the defect are cocaine, drugs, alcohol, Agent Orange, heavy metals or other disruptive materials like radiation. You may not know what genes to change to correct the defect, but the Creator does.

Make the command, *'Creator of All That Is, show me what needs to be done to correct this problem. Now let it be changed. Thank you! It is done. It is done. It is done.'*

For every defective gene, there is always a matching defective gene since they come in pairs. There will always be at least two. Say, *'Creator of All That Is, show me the defective match and change it as well.'*

Witness as the Creator makes the rearrangement, and then the work is done.

If you see this,

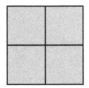

which a visualization of the 'clip', it means the defect was caused by a feeling, and it is the memory causing the body's defect.

Make the command: *'Creator of All That Is, it is commanded that the defective clips be removed, cancelled and sent to God's light and replaced with a proper substitute of a positive feeling, memory, body and future body. Thank you! It is done. It is done. It is done.'*

You will witness the four parts of the clip and any other affected clips as well. It will appear as if you are watching pages of a Rolodex flying off and being replaced. The process happens very quickly. If it is too quick and you feel you haven't seen it all, you may ask for a replay, or for the process to slow down. You must witness the action until the changes on all chromosomes on all four levels are done: the feeling, memory, body and future body:

The first part of the clip is the feeling.
Observe as the defective emotional energy of this portion is pulled and sent to God's light. Observe the new energy coming in from the Creator and replacing the old.

The second part of the clip is the memory.
Next, observe the defective memory portion of the clip being pulled and sent to God's light. Witness the new energy coming in from the Creator and replacing the proper memories for the situation.

The third part of the clip is the body.

Observe the defective body portion of the clip being sent to God's light. Witness the new energy coming in from the Creator. Observe as the body is trained to accept the changes made to it on a physical level regarding the specific ailment.

The fourth part of the clip is the future body.

Witness the defective future body of the clip being sent to God's light. Witness the new energy coming in from the Creator. Observe as the new future body is replaced, making sure that the body does not regenerate the old programme.

The four-part clip will also have a counter or matching defect. Make an identical command process in the same way. Say, *'Creator of All That Is, show me the defective match and change it as well.'* Witness the Creator making the rearrangement, and the work is done.

Any time that you do belief work on a person, you are doing a form of gene replacement on them. If you reach and remove enough of the bottom issues from a client, then the physical issue will be healed as well. All things are connected and interrelated.

Remember, gene replacement is easy to do. You simply witness the processes being done. Most changes happen so quickly that only a flash of light is seen.

You should follow up this process with belief work. Belief work alone can heal the body; it is the key.

CHANGING GENETIC PROGRAMMES FOR AGEING

The people who call me for readings do so for different reasons. Some call to be healed, others for advice, still others for validation and so on. Some of these people are perfectly healthy and they want to remain healthy. For instance, an elderly gentleman called for a reading. When I went into his space I could see that his body was very healthy and as I spoke to it, it told me that it was years younger than it actually was. I did a full body scan but I could not find anything wrong with his body. I told him that he was perfectly healthy and enquired as to why he had asked for a reading. He told me that he knew that he was healthy and he took very good care of himself. For years he had been eating a particular kind of clay that had a high mineral content to promote good health. The reason that he called was because he wanted to change his genetic programmes for ageing. I paused for a moment, and then I thought, 'Why not?' I asked him if he would accept the consequences. When he agreed, I went up to the Creator of All That Is and made the command that his genetic programmes be released and sent to God's light. This is the process that I witnessed:

THE PROCESS FOR CHANGING GENETIC PROGRAMMES FOR AGEING

1. Centre yourself in your heart and visualize going down into Mother Earth, which is a part of All That Is.

2. Visualize bringing up energy through your feet, opening each chakra to the crown chakra. In a beautiful ball of light, go out to the universe.

3. Go beyond the universe, past the white lights, past the dark light, past the white light, past the jelly-like substance that is the Laws, into a pearly iridescent white light, into the Seventh Plane of Existence.

4. Make the command: *'Creator of All That Is, it is commanded that gene work be facilitated on [person's name]. Thank you! It is done. It is done. It is done.'*

5. Go into the person's space into the pineal gland, to the master cell.

6. Make the command: *'Creator of All That Is, it is commanded that all genetic programmes in [person's name] for ageing and getting older be pulled and cancelled, sent to God's light, replaced with the programme of "I am young and ageless, forever regenerating" for all present and future bodies, to be replaced all through the body. Thank you! It is done. It is done. It is done. Show me.'*

7. Witness the process. Stay in the person's space until it is finished.

8. As soon as the process is finished, rinse yourself off and put yourself back into your space. Go into the Earth, pull Earth energy up through all your chakras to your crown chakra and make an energy break.

After this process, the person may feel unwell for a few days, as the body will go through a detoxification process. To avoid this, calcium-magnesium and chelated zinc may be used.

28

VIANNA'S INTUITIVE ANATOMY

This chapter has excerpts from the *Intuitive Anatomy Class Manual*. In the Intuitive Anatomy class it is taught that each system of the body can hold emotions and programmes caused by abuse and other negative influences. Each of the body's systems is explored in the class, along with the psychic energetic influences of each and the negative beliefs that are likely attached to every system.

These are the first and last chapters from the class, explaining the aspect of parasitic influences and the advanced body scan.

MICROBES AND OTHER TOXIC INFLUENCES IN THE BODY

As we study the body systems, we will repeatedly mention disease-causing toxins and microbes. All of these microbes and toxins influence the body and are drawn to you by different *beliefs*.

PARASITES

It is essential to recognize that a person who is infested with parasites is influenced on more than a physical level. Parasites are drawn to the thought processes that block our development on all levels: physically, emotionally, mentally and spiritually. They crave what they need and relay these requests to us, demanding that we eat certain foods. They also relay feelings to us to ensure their own survival, particularly as they die off, when they relay feelings of 'I am dying' to the host, releasing this feeling into the system and causing the host to believe that they are dying. This is generally in response to a parasitic cleanse that the human host is taking.

Feelings and emotions such as 'I must allow others to take advantage of me' and 'I must allow people to suck me dry' are a magnet to parasites. People with parasites may not know how to say 'no'. They have self-esteem issues. When we do belief and feeling work, we are freed from the programmes that attract parasites.

The next step in the process is to free ourselves from parasites of all kinds, such as certain people in our lives. As we remove, replace and add feelings from the Creator of All That Is with the belief work, we will gain the strength to expel many of the micro-parasites from the inner body and expel the human variety from the outer body of our paradigm. Parasites cannot survive in or around a body that doesn't have programmes that will attract them. The fewer limiting beliefs you have, the more balanced the physical pH balance is, creating a healthier body and thus making the body an unhealthy place for parasites.

There are approximately 670,000 *known* parasites. Some parasitical bacteria help digest food and it is normal to have these in the body. For this reason, we do not intuitively command that *all* parasites leave the body.

When someone is grinding their teeth, it is a physical indication of parasites in the body. A parasitic cleanse is in order. This can be done in two ways: by removing and replacing the beliefs that hold parasites to you or by actually taking a parasitic cleanse. Truly, both may be in order, for as a parasitic cleanse is done, feelings and emotions will come up to be cleared.

All meat and vegetables have some parasites. Raw walnuts are one of the most infested foods. Regardless of what you eat, however, the more balanced your beliefs systems are, the fewer parasites you accumulate. Remember, some of these belief systems may be genetic in nature.

If a person has heavy metal poisoning, they seem to have an abundance of parasites. This is undoubtedly due to the weakened condition caused by the heavy metals and the peculiar feelings and emotions that these substances create when in the body.

TAPEWORMS

People come into contact with tapeworms when eating beef, sea food and pork. They can be contracted simply by walking barefoot outside. Once in the body, they attach into the sides of the host's colon, where they steal nutrients. The first indication of a tapeworm is that the host becomes very thin then gains weight. The host will feel hungry all the time. The body thinks it is starving and, because of this, holds on to fat.

FLUKES

Flukes look like snails or leeches in the liver.

CLEANSES

Suggested parasitic cleanses for tapeworms and flukes:

ionic copper
walnut/wormwood combination
cloves
oregano oil (this can be hard on the stomach, so put 2 drops in capsules)
noni juice or seeds

Do belief work before starting a cleanse, as this will make the process smoother. Also be aware that during the cleansing process a healing crisis can manifest and carry the memory of any number of past challenges, such as old infections, toxins, trauma from an accident, and so on. These emotions and physical symptoms may feel real when in reality they are only phantoms of the past.

EXERCISE

Practise entering someone's space to observe their microbes and heavy metals.

HUMAN PROGRAMMES FOR MICROBES AND PARASITES

'I have the Creator's definition of how and when to say "no".'
'I know what it *feels like* to be listened to.'
'I understand what it *feels like* to be heard.'
'I know what it *feels like* to live without being constantly angry.'
'I know what it *feels like* to live without allowing people to suck me dry.'
'I know how to live without allowing people that I love to take advantage of me.'
'I understand what it *feels like* to live without being overwhelmed.'
'I know how to live without being miserable.'
'I know how to interact with others.'

These are just ideas to work on. Follow up this list by doing further belief and feeling work. Remember, every individual is different, so ask the Creator of All That Is what the person you're working with needs to heal.

Θ *It is imperative that you listen to the Creator to see what the person you're working with needs. Remember to listen to the person that you're working with and to dig to the bottom issues.*

HERBAL AND DIETARY SUGGESTIONS FOR PARASITES AND MICROBES

The body needs to be slightly alkaline with a ph of about 7.2 to 7.4 to resist parasites, *Candida*, bacteria and other challenges. It is equipped to fight off viruses, bacteria and parasites, but if it gets out of balance, the immune system is stressed and these entities can get out of control.

Herbal parasitic cleanses should be used only in the spring, not in winter, because then the body is in a rest period. Doing parasitic cleanses constantly can be hard on the body. If it is found that a herbal cleanse is needed, follow this process: *ten days on, five days off, ten days on, five days off, ten days on and five days off*, so that all the eggs that are hatched by the parasite during the process are destroyed.

If you do a parasitic cleanse, it is best to balance it with an alkaline diet so that the process is not so emotional.

The feelings you will experience during a cleanse may not be your own. Feelings like 'I'm going to die' are coming from the consciousness of the parasites and worms that are dying.

Ridding yourself of physical parasites also helps you to let go of emotional parasites and 'energetic' parasites, such as waywards, spiritual hooks, etc.

Seek advice from a healthcare professional before using a cleanse of any kind.

Herbs and Minerals for a Cleanse
   Wormwood-walnut extract: Not for people with diabetes.
   Ionized copper: A very good parasitic cleanse; good for tapeworms.
   Cayenne pepper
   Oregano oil: Put it in a gel cap before consuming.
   Ginger
   Garlic
   Olive leaf extract: Kills yeast as well.
   Fresh juice: 2 carrots, 1 stick of celery, ½ beetroot, little garlic, pinch of ginger. Keeps you clean.
   Noni for pets: 10 days on, 5 days off, as explained above.
   Thyme: Thyme kills parasites in drinking water. One tablespoon of Listerine contains enough thyme to clear parasites that are consumed with water, as well as salmonella.
   Charcoal: Clears giardia and other parasites.
   Colloidal silver: Clears parasites and *Candida*, but taking it all the time is not recommended.
   Platinum: Clears all kinds of parasites and *Candida*.

Do not kill parasites using ThetaHealing. The die-off will create an over-abundance of waste products and dead parasites, causing the person to fall ill. In many instances, pulling and replacing the beliefs that draw and hold parasites will be enough to pass the parasites from the system.

FUNGUS

Fungus infections affect all organs of the body. For example, some sinus infections are caused by it. Mould problems at home and work are common and should be taken care of immediately, before they can create health problems. Black mould in houses is only now beginning to be recognized by public officials for the health hazard that it is.

If someone has a fungus infection, they should consider removing white flour and sugar from their diet and assume an alkaline diet.

Fungus projects programmes of 'I'll do it later'. Through this projection, the person thinks these feelings of procrastination are their own thoughts.

Dead and dying fungus is seen intuitively as a black cloudy substance.

All fungus is tied to resentment issues. Clear the issues and the fungus will go away.

Some Herbs for Fungus
  tea tree oil (use topically only)
  noni
  eucalyptus is anti-fungal/antibacterial (use topically only)
  olive leaf extract

CANDIDA

Many people have *Candida* problems and should consider a balanced alkaline–acid diet. Acidity tends to increase with age and too much of it will explain osteoporosis and the loss of teeth. On the other side of the coin, too much alkalinity will also create a favourable environment for *Candida*.

Candida craves what it needs to survive in the body. It is a problem when a person is too critical or resentful of themselves or others.

It is not advised to intuitively command all the yeast in a person's body to die. The body needs a certain amount of yeast to function.

Intuitively, yeast looks like a dusty, misty or cloudy energy in the body.

An over-abundance of yeast in the body can cause weight gain in some people. Yeast in the colon affects the sinuses.

BACTERIA

Bacteria that are causing challenges in the body can become beneficial when the body is alkaline balanced. Bacteria only become detrimental when the body is out of balance.

Bacteria are easy to get rid of intuitively. Do not command all bacteria in the body to be gone, as some are beneficial.

Guilt issues hold bacteria in the body. Of course, you can always ask the Creator to take care of it and to show you what beliefs are involved.

VIRUSES

Worthiness issues hold viruses in the body. Many people are immune to viral and other sexual diseases when they feel good about themselves and refuse to accept the disease. This may not have anything to do with how the person feels about sex, but rather with how they feel about themselves at the time.

Every virus has the ability to change quickly and mutate to something different in order to survive.

The older the virus is, the smarter it is. Younger viruses, such as AIDS, are not very developed, since they kill their host.

Through the symbiosis between host and virus, the virus will learn to project thoughts to the host to prolong the duration of its life, attempting to get them to stop taking medication that is killing the virus, for example. If you suspect this, ask the Creator what is truly going on in the situation.

VIRUSES SHARE BELIEFS WITH THE HOST

Viruses have the ability to tap into human group consciousness and are drawn to a particular person because they share the same programmes. So we attract diseases to us in the same way that we attract people to us – through parallel belief systems. When we have the same belief system as a virus, bacterium, yeast or fungus, it is attracted to us and attaches itself to us.

In the grand scheme of life we are drawn to one another's negative attributes rather than positive qualities. In a similar way, viruses are drawn to the negative attributes of a person, because negativity makes a person weak physically, mentally and spiritually.

Take a good look at yourself. Do you attract the human equivalent of parasitic energies? I know this is a broad concept and a bold statement, but let me tell you a story.

When I first started to do healings seriously, in the early stages of belief work, I worked with a woman who had herpes. She periodically came in for a healing to clear it, but it wouldn't permanently go away. Every time I did a healing on her, I witnessed Creator sending a tone into her body. This *tone*, or perhaps I should say *vibration*, would put the virus into remission for a while, but then it would come back. And then she would come in for another healing.

During a reading, the Creator told me to witness the beliefs that were being released from the woman were being changed on the herpes virus as well, instead of treating it as if it was a separate entity. So I witnessed the feeling programme of 'I am worthy of God's love' come in. Then I witnessed the *feeling* of God's love come in and instilled the virus with the same feeling. I pulled and replaced more belief systems around and in the virus. As I did so, I watched the virus change into something completely different and leave the body. The woman went to the doctor and was tested to see if the herpes had gone. The tests all came up negative for herpes and it has never come back.

In some instances, viruses are held and hidden on different belief levels. When you are in a belief work session with a client you may find that they have a virus.

Remember that a virus is an alien invader in every cell. Psychically and microscopically, it may look like a robot. Many intuitives will claim that the virus is an alien invader, but *anything* that is alien to the body will come up as an alien invader.

At one time, I used a tone or vibration to destroy viruses. This tone came from the Sixth Plane in marriage with the Seventh. If you want to do this as a process, you go up to God, and then, through God, go to the Sixth Plane, which is where you get the specific tone to send through the body, then move the tone up or down to match the vibration and mutation of the virus. You can also command a bacteria or virus to assume a form that is harmonious to the body, or command the body to be in perfect balance and harmony then move the immune system up. This will change the microorganisms into another harmless form.

To guard ourselves from viruses we change the beliefs that are drawing them to us and then mutate the virus with belief work at the same time. This changes the belief system of the virus so that it does not have to attack us to survive, thus transmuting it to a life form harmless to the host. Since microbes have a group consciousness, all we need to do is to change our group consciousness so that the microbes will have no need to be drawn to our emotions.

We do not want to make viruses our enemy and command that they be gone, since viruses could be the best way to administer medication. Rather, we should witness a virus changed to a form that is harmless.

A virus goes through the cell wall and uses our DNA or RNA to replicate itself, so it can get to the nucleus of the cell, which is a place where I made a discovery. There is some kind of micro-plasma organism that attacks the mitochondria and causes sickness. The mitochondrion has its own DNA and this must also be worked on as well. This is present in everyone that I have seen who has muscular dystrophy.

INTUITIVE REMEDIES

VIRUSES AND BACTERIA HELD ON THE BELIEF LEVELS

Herpes and hepatitis look like little robots when seen intuitively, so it is good to remember that what you are seeing is not aliens, but rather viruses, a different type of invader.

Check to see if the person believes that illness is a punishment or has programmes of 'I should be ill'.

A virus has a belief system of four levels, the same as humans. Ask the Creator of All That Is what feelings to instil so that it will change to a form harmless to the host.

MICRO-PLASMA

Micro-plasma is a cross between a virus and a bacterium. If you find this, work on worthiness and guilt issues.

NANOBACTERIUM

A nanobacterium is a newly discovered bacterium that grows *very* slowly. It causes plaque in the veins and has a calcium shell. When one drinks homogenized cow's milk the nanobacterium uses the dead calcium in the milk. It utilizes it to shield itself from detection by the body's defence systems.

PRIONS

You may know prions best from mad cow disease, in which a rogue protein grows out of control, attaches to another protein and scrambles the protein chains, thus destroying them and scrambling the brains of a cow. A prion is a protein and most are beneficial in nature. The human brain has many prions, which enable the neurons to function.

When doing a healing for mad cow disease, ask the Creator of All That Is to change the rogue prion and show you. Since most prions are beneficial, do not to command that all prions are removed from the body.

HEAVY METALS

Viruses and bacteria are drawn to heavy metals because of the weakness that they cause in the body. The body is actually made up of heavy metals, such as zinc, calcium and magnesium, but some metals are not meant for it, such as aluminum and mercury. The following heavy metals are poisonous and may be the source of many sicknesses:

Aluminium: There are many different sources of aluminum. Aluminum can be a cause of Alzheimer's and Parkinson's disease.

Fluoride: It makes a person age more quickly and leaves deposits in the body.

Iron: Naturally oxidizes in the body. High levels are poisonous.

Lead: Causes depression, insanity, cancer and immunological diseases.

Manganese: Manganese is needed to regulate sugars in the body, but too much can make you go crazy. Psychopathic killers have very high levels in their brain.

Mercury: Mercury makes you depressed and can cause many cancers. It may bind to other heavy metals in the body. Ask the Creator of All That Is to show it to you. Any amount is poisonous. Selenium, coriander or pectin pulls out mercury from the body. These substances bind to the mercury in amalgam fillings and leech out mercury from the fillings. For this reason, it is suggested to take out amalgam fillings first, then do the cleansing. See reference chart on page 308.

Silver: Naturally oxidizes in the body. High levels are poisonous. Overuse of colloidal silver will turn the skin blue.

Heavy Metal Toxicities

Metal	Effect	Found in	Remedy
aluminium	Alzheimer's disease dementia kidney dysfunction senility tumours	antiperspirants some antacids baking powder buffered aspirin toothpaste	cayenne pepper pumpkin seeds red cabbage
cadmium	cancer cardiovascular disease	batteries coffee (traces) paints tobacco white bread (traces)	amino acids calcium chelated zinc
lead	allergies fatigue irritability lack of willpower MS nervous disorders neurological dysfunction tooth decay	fungicides old hair dyes old paint old water pipes tin cans tobacco	basil camomile tea red cabbage rosemary vitamin C vitamin E

If you are in a person's space doing a body scan and you see shiny flecks in their body, it may mean that they have heavy metals there. Calcium, magnesium, zinc, alpha lipoic acid (ALA), omega 3, co-enzyme Q10 and lots of greens have been found to take unwanted heavy metals out of the body. Cleanse the body by asking the Creator how to clear them in the highest and best way. When you detoxify from heavy metals, you pull out old memories attached to them.

The healer should not command all heavy metals from the body to be gone, given that we are made of heavy metals such as calcium and zinc. They are a vital part of our molecular structure. It is best to ask the Creator of All That Is what to do, since everyone is different and toxins should be pulled out of the body at a rate tailored to the individual.

CHEMICAL SENSITIVITY

Chemical sensitivity is a severe problem for many people. Our bodies are becoming overloaded with synthetic chemicals.

The worst culprit, and the most prevalent, is formaldehyde. This is an industrial chemical manufactured from methanol, natural gas and some of the lower petroleum hydrocarbons found widely in the urea formaldehyde foam insulation used in homes and mobile homes.

SOME SOURCES OF FORMALDEHYDE (TRACES)

adhesives
air fresheners
antiperspirants
carpets
cellophane
cleaning solutions
contraceptive creams
cosmetics
dentifrices
detergent soaps
disinfectants
dry-cleaning chemicals
dyes and dyed fabrics
enamel and latex paints
fabric softeners
facial tissues
fertilizers
foam insulation

germicidal products
hairsprays and other hair products
mouthwashes
nail polish
newsprint
pesticides
plastic
plywood
polishes
shampoos
synthesis of some vitamins,
    especially A and E
synthetic fibres
tampons
toothpaste
wallboard
waxes
wood veneer

WHAT CAN CAUSE AN OUT-OF-BALANCE STATE

Electromagnetic Pollution
- communication frequencies
- electrical appliances
- power lines
- telephones
- transformers

Environmental Pollution
- acid rain
- carbon monoxide
- chemical factories – pesticides, plastics, solvents
- crop spraying – fungicides, herbicides, pesticides
- mycotoxins – cryptosporidium
- refineries
- waste treatment plants

Magnetic Fields: Direct Impact
- aircraft
- bed frames
- belt buckles
- bra underwires
- cars
- dental work
- hairpins
- jewellery
- spectacles
- steel buildings and structural beams

Toxic Ingestion
- *drinks:* artificial sweeteners, refined sugar
- *drugs:* alcohol derivatives, phenol, synthetic carrying agents
- *food:* harmful chemicals, preservatives and enhancers

Toxic Substance Radiation
- carpets
- foam rubber
- household cleaners
- pesticides
- plastics

polyurethane
synthetic fabrics
upholstery

HIDDEN PLACES OF MAGNETIC FIELDS AND TOXIC SUBSTANCE RADIATION

In the Workplace
carpets
lighting
machinery
office equipment
power tools
steel buildings
telephones
wallboard

In the Home
bedding
carpets and padding
curtains
electrical appliances
electricity in walls and floors
fabrics
foam padding
kitchen cleaners
lights
mattresses
upholstery
walls

For alleviating difficulties stemming from chemical and heavy metal poisoning a person should first check with a doctor, as there are effective means available to deal with these problems.

DOCTORS AND DIAGNOSIS

While on the subject, it is worth mentioning that in Western society most doctors and patients do not realize how much power we give our doctors. We wait with bated breath on every word the doctor says and believe what we are told, since in our society the doctor knows all. Proper discernment regarding what we are told by our doctor is important, as is the knowledge that there is always an alternative – there are other opinions, and other doctors. Doctors are like us, with positive and negative attributes, and in the end it is always our decision whether or not to accept the opinion of a healthcare provider. Be particularly careful of accepting negative statements from a doctor as the ultimate truth.

On the flip side of the coin, there is the story of a man in hospital dying of a mysterious malady. None of the doctors could diagnose the challenge that was affecting the man, much to the consternation of the patient. One day, a surgeon visited him while making his rounds with a group of interns in tow. After looking over the sick man's chart and talking with him for a bit, the surgeon turned to leave. As he did so, he turned to the interns and said, '*Morto.*' Strangely, after that, the man began to improve. He improved so much so that he got up and left hospital. When asked by a friend the reason for his recovery, he answered, 'I finally found out what I had.' It seems that he interpreted '*Morto*' as a diagnosis on the part of the doctor, and now he could finally put a name to his challenge, all fear of the unknown was gone, and the challenge with it. What the man didn't know was that *morto* is Latin for 'dead' or 'death'. The surgeon was indicating to his students that the man was as good as dead. Just imagine what would have happened to the man if he had understood Latin! This is just one instance of how much power we give to our heathcare providers.

29

SECRETS OF THE INTUITIVE READING SESSION

The structure of a session is generally as follows:

1. Ask permission to enter the person's space.
2. Do a scan of the body. It can take a while to work through all the systems of the body, so ask for the major challenges in that person.
3. If it is necessary, witness the Creator healing as needed.
4. See and speak with the person's guardian angels/guides.
5. Ask the person, 'If there is anything that you would change in your life, what would it be?'
6. Begin using the belief work to dig to find what feelings may need to be taught and what beliefs may need to be released.
7. Have the person ask you questions. Answer the questions and give the person guidance.
8. Give a future reading last because the belief work changes the future.

This is a simplified structure for an otherwise intricate process. A Theta reading is like the music of wind through the leaves and it plays a different melody each time, in each person. The following sections are a guide to the different music being played in the body reading.

THE PRINCIPLES OF THE BODY READING

HOW DO YOU VIEW THE BODY?

Many of my students asked me what *I* was doing when I viewed the inner realm of the body. From listening to them, I knew that I was viewing the body differently from other people. I asked God, 'What am I doing differently from other people?' These are the messages that I received:

The Body Sings

When other people look into the body, they go in looking for something that is *wrong*. They go in with too much stress, tension and emotion. They are trying too hard.

The thing to realize is that the body is wonderful, even magical. When you look into the body and see a single cell, you should listen to how it sings its tiny song of harmony with the rest of the body. All parts of the body, from the smallest cell to the largest organ, sing and resonate with one another with beautiful vibrations. When there is something wrong with an organ, you will hear that it doesn't sing 'true' and sends the wrong signals to the other organs. Learn to listen to these vibrations and their signals. If you are in a person's space in a reading and you hear an organ singing out of tune with another, perhaps the body is out of tune or the organ has a challenge in it. You should then investigate what is amiss.

When you look in the body, remember *it is alive*, so it will never look exactly as an anatomy model would. The colours are far more vibrant and beautiful than any anatomy model.

Go in with Love

The best thing to do when we scan the body is to project the feeling of *love* to it. The body talks to me and tells me what's wrong. I don't go in with stereotypes, I don't hate the viruses, I just talk to the body. I ask it, 'What's going on?'

When I was first doing healings I would tell viruses, 'You're not supposed to be there!' I would hear the shocked reply of, 'I'm not?' Viruses like hepatitis C are not mean or vicious.

When you do a body scan, you may not recognize cancer and sickness in the body because the cancer doesn't think it's bad, and bacteria and viruses may hide from you.

The first time I saw a cancer cell I told it that it wasn't supposed to be there. But it talked back to me and said, 'I'm supposed to be here. I'm not wrong and I'm not bad.' It emitted this self-righteous energy. I understood for the first time what it meant to *love* cancer away. Cancer cells can shift back to normal cells if you guide them to do so.

If you go into a virus with hate, you'll feed it with your emotions, especially if the person is carrying sexual herpes. Check yourself for the programmes of 'I hate illness' and 'I hate ill people'. An illness, whether it is due to bacteria, viruses or fungus, is just energy. It serves you and shows you are out of balance. Work on the attachment and how you view the imbalance. A healer gives a disease more of an identity when they are angry at it. I can see viruses hanging off people when they come in, it is as if they're waving to me saying, 'Hi!' I can see them because I'm not afraid of them. I can see sexual herpes right away, and I'm not afraid of it.

Why should you give a disease all that negative energy? Do not acknowledge it with fear or hatred. If you go into the body with fear or hatred, you won't see all that you can witness. Pull and replace any programmes of fear, anger or hatred. When you go through the body remember that you are not alone, you have the best tutor in the world. Just accept the healing and witness it as done.

If you are trying too hard, the person's body will be resistant and will not show itself to you. Its immune system will be activated and attempt to figure out what's going on. So go in to the body as gently as a feather floating on the breeze. We need to accept that the body is amazing. When you go into it, create the feeling of magic! If you relax and let that feeling flow, you'll be surprised to see how right on you are.

Download the 'knowing' of these programmes:

'Miracles happen every day.'
'The body is a miracle.'
'I will not give in to fear, anger or hatred.'

The Feeling of Vitamins

Practise *feeling* vitamins by taking small doses of them. As you get used to the feeling of them in your own body you will gain the ability to feel and see them in someone else's space. For instance, practise with vitamin B for a week and see what it feels and looks like by entering your own space to experience the energy of it. Then you will be able to tell what vitamins other people may or may not need.

Medicine

Before you begin the reading, ask the client if they are on medication. Avoid suggesting herbs unless you're licensed to do so. They can counteract medications. Always have your client's doctor check them to see if they need their medication changed. Remember, you're not diagnosing, you're praying.

If someone is on asthma medication or some other types of medication, they will need water to energy test correctly, as some medications dehydrate the body. Ask the Creator to show you what the drugs look like in the person's body.

Breathing

Take slow breaths in and release them very slowly. This will lower your blood pressure and help to create a meditative state. This puts you in tune and deeper in a Theta wave.

Discernment

The skill of a healer is to get into the client's life and space and out of their own for the space of the reading. So you must learn to separate the feelings of the client and your own, so that there is crystal clarity in the reading.

Ego

Remember to permit the Creator the opportunity to do the work in a person's space without your own interference and doubts. You should only witness the Creator doing the healing.

Focus

When someone is sitting in front of you, you may have only a few minutes to troubleshoot the full body. If you have limited time, as is the case in many readings, you must develop the focus to pick out the major challenges in the person. Ask the Creator to show you these.

The Future

When you do belief work on yourself or someone else, you are changing the possible future. It is best for the person to ask questions pertaining to the future directly *after* the belief work is done. However, if belief work has already been done in a session, you will need to wait until a later date to do a future reading, since the future will have been changed with the belief work.

Seek the Belief

When you work with someone, watch their facial expressions and you will see them holding on to programmes. Verbally, they will be argumentative, impatient and in denial. They will say things such as 'I don't know' and 'Just fix it.' When a person does this, the healer must be patient and ask, 'What if you did know?' Wait for them to talk and they will come up with the programme on their own. If they don't want to see something, they won't listen to what you have to say. It is best to wait for them to share with you.

Dysfunctional Programmes

Some of these energies are curses, free-floating memories and old connections to the different planes of existence.

Heavy Metals

When you are in a reading, you will most likely find heavy metals in the bloodstream and in the liver. They might be seen intuitively as strange metallic substances. Do not mistake them for alien implants.

Interconnectedness

For every physical ailment that comes to light there is an emotional, mental or spiritual aspect that is connected to it. All aspects of the person must be healed.

Vision

If an area of the body does not show up as clearly as you would like while you are scanning the body, then perhaps there is nothing in that area that you are supposed to see.

Attachment

Get rid of your attachment to the reading and accept what you see in a person's space. Sometimes the Creator reveals different aspects of people in layers over time. Trust and be patient! The more you practise, the more you will perceive.

Judgement

If a client is irritating you, then it may be necessary to do belief work on yourself to explore why. There is a reason why you are 'triggered'. Honour everyone who comes to be worked on, even if they drive you crazy. The key to this work is to be an enemy to no one. Don't make judgement calls on a person, even if you don't agree with their values.

Instant Healing

When instant healing occurs, you will feel the person's body shift and heal with the Creator's force, then the energy will flash back into your space and both you and the client will feel the energy vibrate through you.

Thought Control

Make sure you are disciplined in your thoughts. You can manifest instantly with focused thought when you become experienced with Theta. Test for negative programmes pertaining to responsibility, confidence and abilities. Be responsible for your thoughts.

Some of the psychic blocks that stop manifestations serve a purpose. What would happen if a two year old could manifest anything they wanted? Perhaps there is a Law of Checks and Balances that filters wild and uncontrolled thoughts and does not allow them to come into reality until we are capable of responsible manifestations.

The Feeling of Disease
Once you have intuitively experienced a disease more than once, you will remember it and recognize it in another person's body. Experience will relieve you of fear and doubt. When you do a healing and you know the specifics of the challenge, you see and heal more effectively.

As healers, we think that some diseases are more difficult to work on than others, but this is only a belief. For instance, children heal faster because their beliefs are not set in stone as yet.

The Creator's Love
Bring the Creator's love into the healing. Healing energy isn't created from nothing. The Creator's *love* is the energy that makes the process work.

If, in a reading, the Creator tells you that 'all will be fine', know that things are likely to be difficult for a while. This is the Creator's way of letting you down easy and tells us all that the Creator's *perspective* is different from our own.

Family
Belief work not only benefits the person but their family as well. As you start doing DNA belief changes on yourself, your family will become closer to you. On some level, you will be obliged to help them. They may come to you for help after you've done the work on yourself. Do not push yourself on them. They will come to you when they are ready. This is the family you picked for yourself when you chose to come to this plane! Take care of yourself first and clean up your body, mind and soul.

The 'Knowing'
Energy testing yourself or someone else regarding a specific disease will not be accurate. The subconscious mind may *believe* that it has the disease, so this is not a good indicator that you (or the other person) actually has the disease.

The true indicator that something is true comes from the inner and outer knowing of the Creator and connecting to the Creator.

It is wise to receive validation of a disease or malady from a doctor.

30

CHILDREN OF THE RAINBOW

In the sections ahead we will be discussing children as they grow and develop into mature adults, from the pre-natal (before birth) stage to 32 years old. This information will concern children in general, but specifically those children referred to as 'Indigo Children', 'Rainbow Children' or 'Children of the New Age'. This text is written to offer a guideline that will enable you to work *on* these children, work *with* these children and see challenges with these children when they are very young.

CHILDREN OF THE NEW AGE

RAINBOW CHILDREN

Since the time of the ancients the world has waited for the Rainbow Children to arrive. Rainbow Children are sensitive and incredibly intuitive children. You feel good when you are around them. They are born with infinite wisdom and the ability to change the world around them. They are extremely loving, adaptable human beings with memories of other times, places and skills. They radiate infinite love and patience.

Rainbow Children influence their environment as well as time to meet the needs of humankind. They have an incredible 'knowing' of right and wrong and know how to shift energy.

INDIGO CHILDREN

You need to understand that the term 'Indigo Children' is often misused. An Indigo is a child ushering in a new age, a new time. It is said that these children are a recent phenomenon, but they have been around for at least 45 years and sometimes longer. When we talk about Indigo Children, we are also talking about the Children of Bronze and Gold; these are all

Children of the New Age. These children have been born frequently since the 1960s; however, they have been coming into the world for many years. The oldest Indigo Child I have ever met was 78 years old.

Indigo Children, as well as Bronze and Gold Children, have certain abilities and traits that make them very sensitive to energy around them. As the Indigo Child starts to mature, they seem to be very hypersensitive. In major decisions an Indigo can become almost flighty. This is because they are born with many traits of an artist.

They are easily confused about what they want to do in life, assuming that they have to pick only one specific career. Indigos often start by holding many jobs in high school. If they attend college, they may change their major many times to experience different areas. They have a well-balanced brain with both male and female energy.

An Indigo Child can be overwhelmed by the energy in a room, but a Rainbow Child converts the energy to goodness. An Indigo Child has incredible intuition and is wonderful at manifesting. However, an Indigo Child can be influenced by negativity, unlike a Rainbow Child, who simply changes it. Indigo Children are now transforming into the vibration of Rainbow Children.

BRONZE CHILDREN

Bronze Children are the scientists of the future; they love to put things together and take things apart. They are continually asking, 'Why?' These are the children who want to grow up and become botanists, microbiologists, quantum physicists and work in other areas of scientific exploration. It is rare that they change their minds.

Bronze Children are focused and determined to find answers. They will be responsible for finding answers for the ozone layer issue and solving the problems with our water. Like Indigo Children, they have traits of love and compassion. They are involved in proving that God and science often go hand and hand. They understand how energy works and that it can be studied.

GOLD CHILDREN

Gold Children are those who come into the world with immense healing and manifesting abilities. They are born healers and they have no doubts concerning the Creator's healing power. Whereas Indigo and Violet Children have healing abilities, Gold Children are adept at creating manifestations and can actually 'see' the problem and repair it. They excel in the area of healing emotions, both physically and genetically.

Even though Gold Children are often artistic, they focus primarily on healing. They choose at a very young age what they desire their life to be. Many Gold Children become doctors, surgeons or medical scientists.

Indigo, Bronze and Gold Children all share artistic talents, scientific abilities, immense healing and visionary abilities. All of them feel love and empathy for others and have an intuitive nature. They are prototypes of the evolution of the human brain. The frontal lobes of these children are extended and operate at a much faster pace. In CAT scans, it has been shown they have extra electrical activity in the frontal lobes.

The differences in these children's DNA make them more immune to diseases as they grow older. When they are small, however, great care must be taken with Indigo and Bronze children, because they are hypersensitive. In some instances they are allergic to substances in their environment, for example yellow and red dyes. Although Gold Children are susceptible as well, eventually they can train their bodies to live anywhere in the world they wish without negative reactions.

Indigo, Bronze and Gold children are evolving into Rainbow Children. They are all intuitive and psychic and have the ability to see guardian angels and obtain knowledge through their crown charka. Some may be interested in the concepts of different religions, expanding the understanding of the 'One Creator' that they already had before coming into this world.

Every human being is born with empathetic (feeling) skills. Starting from the first day of life, the human subconscious picks up thoughts and feelings from others. The human psyche naturally reads and perceives the energy that penetrates its aura. But because these children are extremely intuitive, they are sensitive to the world around them and sense other people's feelings as their own. Unable to sort out and pull away from other people's feelings, they will cry when their mother or father cries and often wonder why people treat each other so harshly. This explains why little children often think that they are not liked, that they have done something wrong or that there is something wrong with them. Guiding the development of their empathetic skills will teach them the difference between their own feelings and someone else's.

New Age Children are extremely loving and, unlike many children, are kind and want everyone to be in harmony. They often feel out of place and can definitely 'feel' vibrations as to whether they are liked or disliked.

It is very difficult for these children to go to school because other children can sometimes be very cruel. It is even more difficult if the teacher has no empathy or is unkind toward the child. These children *must* like their teacher and be encouraged to learn. They are usually more intelligent than the average child. They comprehend quickly, get bored easily and as a result are often misdiagnosed with attention deficit disorder (ADD). Many of these children are put on medication they don't need. I observe parents constantly putting their children on medication when the only thing the child is guilty of is being a child. If that child can sit down and play a video game for two hours, the chances of attention deficit disorder are not high. Also, some parents wait until later in life to have children and are unaware of how little children behave and grow.

The children being born at this time, the Indigo, Bronze, Gold or Rainbow Children, are incredibly wonderful, spiritual, fantastic children. But if they have any slight chemical deficiencies, they can become aggressive. You must realize that if children are aggressive by nature they may not be Children of the New Age. I frequently read articles that state that Indigo Children are overly aggressive and that this aggression is normal. This aggression is *not* normal and is *not* typical behaviour for a child.

Since Rainbow Children are incredibly intuitive, in the normal course of events their brain polarity will switch. Brain polarity is extremely easy to reverse; people change their polarity every day. For instance, anytime I do intuitive readings, my polarity reverses. Do not give children medication to change their polarity to normal; the reversal is part of being a New Age child.

These children also have the capacity to step out of their own paradigm. They are able to go into another person's space and understand them. Although they have a love of self, they also have the ability to externalize and see how others around them feel.

CHEMICALS OF THE BRAIN

There is new kind of epidemic ravaging our children; you should be aware of it and be able to recognize it. It isn't a germ and it isn't a poor diet, it is brain damage caused by traumatic experiences. Such damage can affect the development of the brain and can cause problems ranging from aggression to language failure, depression and other mental disorders. It can cause physical disorders as well, such as asthma, epilepsy, high blood pressure, immune deficiency disorders and diabetes. All of these problems increase as people experience environmental stresses including poverty, violence, sexual abuse, family break-ups, drugs, lack of good stimulation and too much of the wrong stimulation. These influences are pouring into the brain through sight, smell, touch and sound. This puts a great deal of importance on parenting, because parenting has a big impact on the way the brain becomes wired.

How do experiences affect the brain? The brain has stress hormones called cortisol and adrenaline. These hormones are designed to respond to psychological and physical danger; they prepare the body for fight or flight. Normally these transitions from one emotion to the other are fairly smooth. They are important survival skills that we must learn. When the brain is continually stressed as a child, however, even in the foetal or newborn stage, these hormones become overactive. If this stress persists, it will cause the foetal development to change. Persistent stress will take a directive from the genes and change it dramatically, causing a network of brain cells to be distorted and imprinting the brain with misguided signals. These signals can cause epileptic seizures, because instead of a clear signal between the cells, there is a different one. These children may have a depressive episode instead of a happy thought. They have surges of rage instead of willingness to compromise.

Much of this occurs even before birth and such damage can hardly be detected in the beginning, but you'll see it as the child grows. If a pregnancy is difficult or if the baby is not wanted, it will perceive these emotions. The baby knows from the moment it is conceived if it is wanted or not wanted. If a pregnancy is stressful, the baby will learn to create chemicals that cause it to go into fits of rage or anger or depression. These things can be changed as the tiny baby begins to grow. They can be changed by loving parents and kind words, but it takes time. The problem that faces our society is the fact that many people are not approaching marriage in a responsible way. This is because part of the frontal lobe doesn't develop until the mid-twenties.

Young mothers are often not educated and are unaware how to take care of their own children. There is a pheromone that is released from the mother to the child that bonds that child to the mother forever. If the mother doesn't have that pheromone receptor, she will not have the instinct to protect the child.

The human condition is magic when it begins. If a baby is conceived in love and talked to throughout the gestational period, its brain will develop normally. But if it is unwanted at conception or under high stress throughout the gestational period, it will emerge into the world ready to fight or run at the first indication of trouble. Later, when the child starts school and faces correction from a teacher, that correction will be taken as a personal affront and the child will fight the criticism instead of accepting it as a loving, learning experience.

Secondly, there are many parents in this day and age that are not able to provide financially for their own families. In many instances this is partly due to poor education and lack in their own homes when they were growing up. I don't mean to imply that you necessarily have to be rich to have a child, but it would certainly be nice if a child born into the world did not have to go hungry. Poverty is such a problem today. Children who are born into homes where they are not wanted as well as into poverty face problems from the outset.

Thirdly, there is the lack of commitment from the parents. By not being committed to each other the parents start this whole scenario without a base structure. Since there is no commitment, one of them will eventually leave and the child will feel loss and abandonment.

With the combination of being unwanted, growing up in poverty and having non-committal parents, a child may face tremendous difficulties in just coping with daily life. These are important things for you to understand.

As the foetus grows and develops in the womb, it remembers everything that is going on. The brain is constantly developing neurons as the child is growing, and if a loving, caring environment is being experienced, it will develop normally. However, if it is under stress, it has a higher likelihood of illness. It will be more prone to a broad range of diseases and have a higher probability of structural problems in the neurons, causing society to need to build more prisons.

Aggression is not necessarily a bad thing. It has enabled us to compete for food, shelter, mates, status, etc. It's actually very universal, and every vertebrate on the Earth has used it to gain survival and reproductive advantages. On some level, aggression is an important trait that allows us to stand up for ourselves. Normal aggression has a set point, like body temperature, and it is regulated by brain chemicals. Most people are born with balanced chemicals and this helps them react to situations in a reasonable way. This set point can be changed, however, by different conditions arising in the brain. Some of this can be genetic – some of us have a tendency to carry genes that make us more aggressive or violent than others. Many people will argue with this and say that we aren't our genes and that genetic programming does not influence our behaviour, but in reality it does.

NORADRENALINE AND SEROTONIN

To understand some of the brain's chemicals, we'll start with the basics.

Serotonin, a neurotransmitter involved in the transmission of nerve impulses, is the brain's master. It is the modulator of all our emotions. It keeps our aggression in line, and when it fails, violence rises.

Noradrenaline is the arousal hormone. Noradrenaline and serotonin have much to do with both hot-blooded and cold-blooded violence. If noradrenaline is turned on high and left there, it will produce violence, murders and 'hot-blooded'-type killings. On the other hand, low levels of noradrenaline cause under-arousal. To get their thrills, people with low noradrenaline levels will take calculated risks, sometimes the kind associated with predatory violence, premeditated and cold-blooded murders and serial killings.

Serotonin and noradrenaline may work separately or together in various combinations to produce a different spectrum of violent activity. At normal levels, serotonin keeps everything that drives the emotions in check. In future we may be able to master the serotonin levels and maintain proper balance in regulating sex, mood, appetite, sleep, arousal, pain, aggression and suicidal behaviour. Such control is exerted though the neo-cortex, the part of the brain that oversees the social part of our life, the memories and judgement. It rests like a controlling harbour of primitive instincts and emotions.

RISKS ASSOCIATED WITH LEVELS OF NORADRENALINE AND SEROTONIN

Noradrenaline

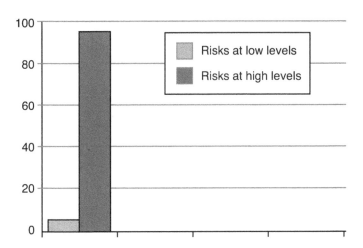

Risks at low levels	*Risks at high levels*
Under-arousal	Over-arousal
Increased tendency toward	Increased tendency toward
pre-meditated or cold-blooded acts	impulsive hot-blooded acts of
of violence	violence
Thrill-seeking	Rapid heartbeat

Please note: This only applies if the serotonin levels are low. Normal levels of serotonin will counteract the above risks.

Serotonin

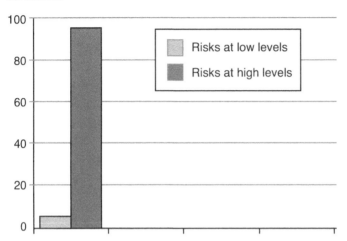

Risks at low levels	Risks at high levels
Depression	Shyness
Suicide	Obsessive-compulsive disorder
Impulsive aggression	Fearfulness
Alcoholism	Lack of self-confidence
Sexual deviance	Unduly dampened aggression
Explosive rage	

Sources: *The AMA Encyclopedia of Medicine, America Heritage Dictionary of Science,* news reports, *Chicago Tribune*/Stephen Ravenscraft and Terry Volpp

INFLUENCES ON BRAIN CHEMICALS

Various things affect both the serotonin and noradrenaline levels. One of these is a difficult family life. For instance, serotonin declines in people who have parents who are alcoholic or drug abusers. Alcohol has been known to provoke aggression and we are finally realizing how much it changes the chemistry of the brain by lowering the serotonin level. Also, one out of every four children in America is being raised by a single parent. This causes great financial distress for the parent, greatly affecting the circumstances at home. Steroids also cause a change in the serotonin levels. Sometimes people experiment with steroids, which throw off all the chemicals in their brain and may lead to too much noradrenaline and aggressive and violent behaviour.

Some people can actually diet themselves into aggression. Low-cholesterol diets may provoke aggressive behaviour. Serious injury of any kind can also cause problems. One of the causes that should never be overlooked is the exposure to lead, lead fuels and paint. Anything that contains lead can cause violent behaviour in people and cause a terrible chemical disruption. On the other hand, mercury will cause such terrible depression that after exposure some people become suicidal. Proper serotonin levels enable us to live our lives in harmony.

Even though serotonin isn't the only neurotransmitter linked to aggression, it is extremely important in our life. Scientists have found that there are 16 different serotonin receptors and know there are probably hundreds more. Many people inherit a gene that makes them more susceptible to low serotonin, but early life experiences can change that.

Living in a household that is more violent than normal will actually make a difference as to whether the serotonin level is low or normal. However, there is an enzyme called monoamine-oxidase #A, which is found in families where the men are prone to violence. These men can become rapists and killers with very little provocation. The defective gene is carried by the x chromosome, but it only shows up in the males. Females have two x chromosomes, which contain one good gene that will always override the bad one. The aggressive gene is certain to be found in every dangerous criminal in prison today.

In a case of too much noradrenaline and not enough serotonin, scientists have actually found a way to partially balance the brain by resetting the serotonin level in the brain with different forms of medication. Of course, you can also reset the serotonin level through healing. Children are so easy to work on in this way, and when the serotonin level is changed, the effects can be noticed immediately.

Medication that will work on altering the serotonin level is helpful in teenage depression and other depression that affects people throughout their life. But as a healer, I offer you the following suggestion: it is vital that you remember that the brain has incredible power to heal itself, and telling the brain what to do will create a magnificent change in people immediately. Going into Theta and programming the brain to do something will change things very quickly.

For a very long time we were helpless when it came to diseases of the brain such as Huntington's, Alzheimer's and Parkinson's diseases. But now we know we can actually change the brain and have it restore itself.

When women go through menopause it causes such a disturbance in the brain that it is not quite sure what's going on. Small amounts of oestrogen at this time can revitalize and rejuvenate the brain. It's essential that you realize that all hormones are very important for the brain. In some instances a person's hormones are out of balance and they've been given serotonin or an anti-depressant by their doctor. But what is the underlying cause? In some cases it is their thyroid that's off, or their adrenals that are having a hard time. We need to ask the Creator what is causing the person's problems. We also need to know how to manipulate parts of the brain.

THE PROCESS FOR NORMALIZING BRAIN CHEMICALS

1. Centre yourself in your heart and visualize going down into Mother Earth, which is a part of All That Is.

2. Visualize bringing up energy through your feet, opening each chakra to the crown chakra. In a beautiful ball of light, go out to the universe.

3. Go beyond the universe, past the white lights, past the dark light, past the white light, past the jelly-like substance that is the Laws, into a pearly iridescent white light, into the Seventh Plane of Existence.

4. Make the command: *'Creator of All That Is, it is commanded that [person's name]'s noradrenaline, serotonin and hormone levels be balanced in the highest and best way as is appropriate at this time. Thank you! It is done, it is done, it is done.'*

5. Move your consciousness over to the person's space. Go into the brain and witness the noradrenaline/serotonin levels as a visualized graph. Witness the noradrenaline/serotonin levels become balanced as is proper for the person.

6. As soon as the process is finished, rinse yourself off and put yourself back into your space. Go into the Earth, pull Earth energy up through all your chakras to your crown chakra and make an energy break.

DRUGS FOR THE BRAIN

In this day and age there are some wonderful drugs for the brain. For instance, there's something called a growth hormone that is fantastic! It actually enables the brain to reproduce and replenish itself. Another growth factor is called GM1 ganglioside. It helps people with Parkinson's by triggering the brain to supply dopamine. In Parkinson's cases the dopamine terminals on the neurons are all damaged and GM1 ganglioside can actually help replace them.

The key to having the brain continue to replenish itself and continue working is the nerve growth factor called neurotrophic. Different factors of this are found in the brain, such as the neurotrophic-3. These neurotrophics are like super nannies of the brain cells. They keep the brain cells nourished and make certain they grow and have a long life. They guard them against any kind of damage and make sure the brain functions properly. If they decline and disappear, the brain will be torn apart by free radicals.

There have been many tests to discover why little children can repair themselves so quickly. The reason they can repair their brain so quickly is because their bodies have not stopped growing yet. When the brain reaches a certain age it actually shuts down different growth factors. When it is young, it can repair damage more quickly. That's why children can recover from strokes faster than anyone else.

31

How Children Develop

FOETAL AND BIRTH STAGE

FOETAL MEMORY

Evidence from foetal learning paradigms of classical conditioning, habituation and exposure learning reveal that the foetus has a memory. The existence of this, in some form, is no longer in doubt.

There are a number of possible reasons why the foetus should have a memory, not perhaps one of the complexity of an adult or even infant, but sufficient to ease the baby's progress in the world after birth. Possible functions that have been discussed are: practice, recognition of and attachment to the mother, promotion of breastfeeding and language acquisition. Further studies are required. For more information, see: Foetal Behaviour Research Centre, School of Psychology, The Queen's University of Belfast, Belfast, Northern Ireland, UK.

SENDING LOVE TO THE BABY IN THE WOMB

From the moment of conception, babies are aware of everything around them. The feelings, emotions and beliefs of the mother are often projected to them. Traumatic thoughts, feelings of not being wanted, of being overwhelmed and other stresses can affect their noradrenaline and serotonin levels. Alcohol and the use of drugs also affect the mental health and physical development of the foetus. Some babies start out as twins, but nature only allows about one third of the twins that are conceived to be born. This sometimes causes severe loneliness in the remaining twin. Attempted abortions also affect an individual.

The 'Sending Love to the Baby in the Womb' exercise is an amazing healing process. You can do this exercise on yourself, on your children and on your parents – realizing, of course, that they have free agency as to whether they accept it or not. With clients, you must have their verbal consent to do this exercise. This exercise can benefit many diseases, such as foetal alcohol syndrome, bi-polar disorder, attention deficit disorder and autism, and may simply eliminate them altogether.

After 'Sending Love to the Baby in the Womb', you will still understand negative emotions, but doing this exercise will reprogram the subconscious from a place of true love.

Don't get caught up in the drama of feelings in this exercise. Stay focused.

THE PROCESS FOR SENDING LOVE TO THE BABY IN THE WOMB

1. Centre yourself in your heart and visualize going down into Mother Earth, which is a part of All That Is.

2. Visualize bringing up energy through your feet, opening each chakra to the crown chakra. In a beautiful ball of light, go out to the universe.

3. Go beyond the universe, past the white lights, past the dark light, past the white light, past the jelly-like substance that is the Laws, into a pearly iridescent white light, into the Seventh Plane of Existence.

4. Make the command: *'Creator of All That Is, it is commanded that love be sent to this person as a baby in the womb. Thank you! It is done. It is done. It is done.'*

5. Now go up and witness the Creator's unconditional love surrounding the baby, whether that baby is you, your own child or your parents. Witness love filling the womb and enveloping the foetus, simply eliminating all poisons, toxins and negative emotions.

6. As soon as the process is finished, rinse yourself off and put yourself back into your space. Go into the Earth, pull Earth energy up through all your chakras to your crown chakra and make an energy break.

Let's start at the beginning. A mother is waiting for her infant to be born. This is a tiny important being, one of God's creations. The baby's brain is developing and the mother talks every day of her love for her baby, knowing that this will influence the child's future life. This little child is now in the womb and is growing very quickly.

A baby can hear the mother quite well by seven months. Of course, sound is muffled by the water surrounding the foetus, but the baby can tell the difference in the sounds and definitely knows the difference in feelings.

When the child is born, the first touch is an incredible experience. Caressing the baby, the mother reaches over with a tender kiss. When she does this, her body makes antibodies for her baby that are needed immediately in the new environment. This happens every time she touches the baby. And when she does so, their DNA connects and communicates. It is incredible to know that the human body is so complicated and so wonderful.

Seemingly magical things start to happen. The baby releases strange pheromones to the mother. The mother feels the change and suddenly becomes like a 'mother bear'. If anyone comes too close and tries to harm that baby, the mother will become very defensive and will protect the baby with her own life. If the pheromones are working correctly, the mother's need to hear the child becomes paramount. She can hear every whimper and every sigh. The new mother is very anxious and very careful to check her baby to make certain that everything is safe and sound. For some mothers it may take a couple of days for this to happen. When it does, they become a little more panicky and more nervous, but soon mother and baby will be settled in with each other and doing just fine. This stage is important, since the child realizes that it's OK to be a boy or a girl.

If the birth has been stressful, the mother should hold her baby more to show her love. This will teach the brain to produce more serotonin and the child will begin to mellow and be happy.

Occasionally, a mother has no receptors to her baby's pheromones and, just as in nature, will try to abandon her offspring or have no emotional attachment. Thankfully, this is rare and can be altered with belief work.

Given lots of love, the child stretches forth to see the world. Scientists tell us that babies cannot see well at first, but every mother will tell you that her baby sees her. Scientists will also tell you that a baby doesn't really smile, that it is just an involuntary muscle response, but every new mother knows that her baby smiles at her.

Every human being is born with empathetic (feeling) skills. The human subconscious picks up thoughts and feelings from others and the human psyche naturally reads the energy that penetrates its aura. Because it is a natural instinct and ability, young children are unaware in the beginning how to discern thoughts and feelings in a room from their own. Guiding children in the development their empathetic skills will teach them the difference between their own feelings and someone else's.

Breast milk is ideal for the baby, at least for the first six months. It will actually change for each feeding to meet the needs of the individual baby. This unique substance cannot be duplicated artificially and contains antibodies that provide immunity against infections.

All the New Age babies sleep better in the presence of others. A little bit of noise in the background actually helps them sleep. It isn't until the third month that a baby can fall into a deep REM sleep. By the sixth month, the ability to sleep for longer periods of time has increased.

An important insight for the new mother and the new father is the fact that they should speak to their baby constantly. The more they speak, the faster the child learns. Children learn almost all of their speaking ability from their parents and those close to the family, not from the television or the computer. The Children of the New Age will suddenly try to begin speaking, making sounds and noises as they play with their new vocal cords as their brain begins to grow and mature. At this particular time, all new babies have twice as many neurons in their brain as a normal adult. Science has acknowledged that a baby will mimic the sounds of 'I love you' at three months old, and seem to know what it means. This is also when the mother will notice that when she is upset, the baby is upset.

Babies will also pretend that they are trying to fly or look as if they are flying. They will often look as though they know everything, as if they are old people trapped in a little body.

INFANCY TO 12 MONTHS

Every child develops at their own rate, but they all go through some specific stages. From infancy to 12 months old is a very important one. The child will learn to walk and talk, get teeth and learn sensory discrimination. Children grow faster during this period than at any other time. The number of brain cells and the number of connections in the brain both increase dramatically.

As the nervous system matures, the child's senses develop quickly. Newborns can distinguish sound and objects when they are close to their face. By three months a baby can distinguish colour and form and can mimic sounds. The child will reach up to grab and hold objects between the thumb and forefinger by four months. At four to six months the baby can sit up for short periods of time without support. Crawling starts between seven and ten months. By 12 months, most infants can stand up alone and can walk with assistance. At 14 months most can walk unassisted. This is true even with New Age children, although they may sometimes walk before they crawl. If this is the case, you must make certain that they crawl or their brain will not develop in the right sequence.

Girls usually try to talk sooner than boys do, and boys usually walk, climb and try to conquer physical obstacles sooner. By the time they are one year old, little boys have learned to crawl and definitely learned to conquer. They are trying very hard to walk, if they are not walking already.

If they are not walking, it will be only a short time before they are. They are very curious and attempt to investigate everything. They learn quickly from taste and seem to put everything in their mouth.

The first words are usually uttered between 12 and 18 months, but not so with the little New Age baby. Many of them can say several words before they are 18 months old. The more you talk to your babies, the faster they will speak, and they can learn to mimic words almost from birth. These are important times when the parent must know that the subconscious does not understand the words 'doesn't', 'not' or 'don't'. Use the word '*no*'. If you tell a baby, 'Don't touch it,' they may think that you said to 'touch it' and will try immediately to touch it. They will look very puzzled as you slap their little hand. Be very careful at these stages because what you say to your child may stay with them for the rest of their life.

One of the most interesting things about New Age children is the fact that they can actually see beings of light standing beside you. Many of them see the guardian angels, guides and visitors that come to them. If encouraged, not to the point of overdoing it but if just left alone, they will keep this ability all of their life. It is only when they are told that they can't see these light beings or that they don't exist that they shut down this ability.

ONE TO TWO YEARS

By the time little girls reach the age of one, they are becoming quite the little conversationalists, and some little boys may be the same. However, although conversation seems to be key for little girls, this is not always the case.

One to two years is the age sometimes referred to as the 'terrible twos'. At about this age children are into everything, playing with pots and pans and experiencing life. The more they can touch and feel, the happier they will be. If they are allowed to play in the dirt and sand, they will be healthier later in life.

By the time they reach the 'terrible twos' they should have an understanding of the word 'no'. This is very important. I have never considered any of my children to be a 'terrible two' child. I've always considered them wonderful!

Up to this point the child has been living by instinct. This instinct is as follows: children know that if they cry, the parents will come and take care of them, and that if they smile and laugh, they will be rewarded. By two years of age, however, they begin to investigate more of the world and show some independence. This is because the brain is developing at a higher rate than before. So it is all quite natural and normal for children to veer off a little at this time.

There is no specific age to toilet train a child. Up until about 15 months a child does not have the actual muscles to control the bladder or the bowel appropriately. Being emotionally ready is an important element. Once children are aware of bodily functions and what society expects, they will learn to potty train almost by themselves. Stress and fear of performance can cause problems, so it is advisable for parents to let children take their time. In some societies it is almost a game.

Little boys seem to have a harder time holding their bowels than do little girls, and most girls will be toilet trained sooner than boys. Little girls do not like to feel wet so they learn very quickly how not be wet. Do not push a child; sometimes children are not ready until they are three years old. It is vital, however, that they are taught the value of hygiene.

Children are also becoming very aware of their sexual organs at this time and soon they will be aware of their sexuality. They should never be made to feel shameful but just be allowed to 'be'.

By the time New Age children are two, they may be telling you stories of the Creator and the things they know. Listen to these children; sometimes they have knowledge beyond what you think.

THREE TO FOUR YEARS

Three and four year olds can actually learn to read quite easily and if you take the time with them, you will be surprised by how much they can learn. Children like to learn in small increments of 30-40 minutes because their brain thinks very quickly. They are also constantly learning through taste and smells and the sensations around them.

Up to the age of three years, children get tired easily and when they get tired, they get grouchy. It's always interesting to watch parents becoming angry with their children for getting too tired. Children should have a chance to rest when they are tired.

From birth to the age of four, the child has twice as many neurons in the brain as they will have when they are an adult. They have learned to think, hear, see, taste and learned to develop with the world around them. Between the ages of three and four they are entering into a new stage in their brain. This gives them a false sense of independence. Suddenly they are questioning your behaviour; suddenly they are questioning what you say.

The three year old getting angry because they were made to do something and the four year old who has decided they are going to tell you to do something – both are normal stages of development. No, your child is not terrible. No, your child does not have any 'problems'. Your child is just four, and four year olds do that; four-year-old children *push*. They can love and kiss you one minute, and the next minute they will attempt to push you and tell you what to do. This is the bossy four year old. Even though some children may start this behaviour before they reach four years, maybe two or three months before they are four, you'll know it when they hit that stage. That lovely little baby you've been holding and rocking for so long has suddenly became a little person – a little pushy, a little bit of a know-it-all, someone who won't listen. You may need to put them in time-out for a little while so they understand that they are not the boss.

At this time it is also important for parents to remember that children are wonderful. It is important to be their friend, but it's critical to be their parent. Being a parent doesn't mean that your child always has to like you. Being a parent means that as your child is developing, you have to use good judgement pertaining to their safety.

It is usually around the fourth year that a child learns to negotiate. Many adults call this *manipulation*, but when the child is older it will be called *negotiation*. For now, you need to demonstrate to your child that there are some problems that can be solved and some bargains that can be made. It is important to teach the word 'no', but if that's all you say then by the time the child reaches adulthood they will not know how to negotiate the world around them.

This is a time when it would be using good judgement to go up and ask the Creator how to solve these problems. Knowing that this is a normal behaviour for four-year-old children will keep you from being hurt, offended and upset when your child talks back. This is when their serotonin and noradrenaline levels are reaching their balance and their little circuits are beginning to work at full bore. This is perfectly normal. They still love you; they are just learning to be more independent. Three- and four-year-old children are very interesting indeed.

FIVE YEARS

You now have a five year old and you're quite proud. You've made it through the three- and four-year-old stage and now your five year old is beginning school. Truly, this will be a very interesting experience for them.

Although they will be excited, sometimes it will be very emotionally difficult for them. Giving them positive support such as 'I know you can do it', 'I have faith in you', 'You are wonderful' and 'What an incredible being you are' can help them. Having them be around other children before they start school is also very wise. If they become acquainted with other children at an early age, they will understand how to get along with them when they first start school. One of the biggest mistakes made by parents is keeping their children separate from other children. When they have to enter the school situation it will be very difficult if they have not met other children. Teaching children to learn to negotiate with other children also teaches them to keep their serotonin levels up.

SIX YEARS

By the time children reach six years old they experience another mental stage of development. This one is very much like the four-year-old stage, only a little deeper. The tendency is toward a more independent nature. They really begin to push you and question your decisions. Even though a four year old may seem difficult and at times hurt your feelings, a six year old may often want their own way and there will be times when they are not allowed to have it. A six year old can be a bit demanding and often test your limits to see how much they can get away with. This is when you need to understand that this too is a natural stage of development. Understand that you are there to help your child grow and make these changes. Prepare yourself for your six year old and you will be just fine.

SEVEN AND EIGHT YEARS

Through the ages of seven and eight, the child will normally mellow out and become a little bit easier to handle. This is a normal result of the development of the brain. By now the lobes of the brain have begun to have different sensory perception.

Up until now children have been a tiny bit near-sighted. Make sure that you are aware of this, so that when you decide to take them to get their eyes checked you are not in shock to find out they are a little near-sighted. Their eyes are developing as they go. They can see blues and greens and all the different colours of the spectrum, but green appears a deeper, bluer green now than it does later. Colours change as children grow, so understand that colours may not be exactly the same for your child as they are for you.

By now, they're learning to read and write. This is a time to watch these wonderful children, since many of them have what is called a genius gene. Genius genes are often right next to what is called the dyslexic gene, and often they may invert their letters. Be patient with your child as they learn to read so they are confident with their reading and enjoy it. Reading to them will help them explore the wonderful world of learning.

NINE YEARS

I used to think that there had to be a reason why some churches baptized their children at age eight – it was to prepare them for the age of nine!

Nine is an interesting stage; it is when a child's brain starts to kick in and they become even more independent. This is also when their body is beginning to change and they are remarkably different from that little baby you brought home. This is what I refer to as the 'hell' age. It is the age when they seem to know everything, want to take over everything and get very emotionally upset over everything. This is the onset of new hormonal changes in the brain that alter how the child functions. It is an important time when you need to inform people around you that your child will be back in just a few months. Just be patient, kind and loving but firm through this stage of development.

The love that we receive from our children fills our cup with joy and happiness as we watch them grow and mature. As they make changes in their life, we take offence. We get hurt when they talk back to us and some of the things they say to us hurt us deeply. Be aware, these are baby humans being moulded. We need to be patient, but we also need to be firm. A parent must remember that their child will probably be OK at 10 and will most likely be fine by 11 years old.

As they grow toward adulthood, children learn things very quickly. If encouraged to learn when they are small, it will become a habit and they will continue to learn forever. It is also important that you keep them involved athletically as much as possible to keep them from going astray, so to speak. It is also great for children to be involved in music.

TEN TO FOURTEEN YEARS

It is important from the age of nine onward to watch your children when they are around their friends. Peer pressure is very difficult at this stage and it gets more difficult as they turn 13 and 14. It is vital that you give your children the right guidelines regarding their physical bodies.

The children of alcoholics will often experience dips in their serotonin levels at this time and their noradrenaline levels will start to surge. These are the important ages when you need to watch your children, because the body craves what it needs. When people start craving alcohol, the body is trying to compensate for a lack of serotonin and dopamine. I repeat, this is the time to monitor children closely. Provide them with a good healthy diet, supplement their diet with vitamins and minerals and try to help them so they don't fall into the vicissitudes of addiction. Addictions are very difficult for New Age children. This is when you must trust your intuition and not your emotions. This is a gamble and your psychic energy needs to be on form.

No parent wants to think that their children are in the liquor cabinet sipping alcohol, but chances are good that if they have access to it they will experiment with it, so you need to be on guard for it. This doesn't mean that all children will experiment; nevertheless, you need to be wise and not close your eyes to the possibility. Help your children make wise decisions.

When a New Age child is 10, their feelings will be hurt very easily. If they are teased by other children, they will sometimes just allow it. Teach them they need to stand up for themselves and that it is not wrong to do so. Explain to these children that being intuitive will be important for their survival as the New Age develops. As more children naturally become more intuitive, it will be more accepted. You also must teach them that some people can't recognize or accept their great talents and abilities. This is unfortunate, and we should have empathy for these people; however, prepare your child for these conditions. Some people shut down these beautiful, intuitive children and they are doing them a great injustice by attempting to program them into being something different.

Many of these intuitive children have reactions to yellow and red dye. The parents mistake the symptoms for attention deficit disorder, but this is not the case. Some of these children are actually very brilliant and have no such disorder. Some are allergic to processed white sugar. Processed white sugar is very hard on these children since their chakras are wide open. In addition, their brain development and psychic senses are much more developed than they were in children 10 to 15 years ago. These children are super-hyped, super-sensitive children. If you can keep them away from white flour and white sugar, yellow dye and red dye, you will find they will grow quite normally and will be less likely to become out of control.

It is my belief that in the education of our children, the children may not be the individuals who should change. It just might be their teachers who need to change. Some of our teachers have been teaching for a long time. They are bored and really have no interest in the children. Remember when you were at school? However, in observing the teachers of today, I think you will find that a great many of them have improved their teaching and are changing their attitude about many things. It is important that you find good teachers so that your student can learn and grow.

Some parents have decided to home school their children to keep them safe from the dangers that fill our schools, which is understandable. At the same time, however, they are not allowing their children to interact with children other than those in their own surroundings, and their children will someday have to live in the outside world. If you are home schooling your children, please make sure that they have plenty of time with other children so they can learn to adapt and adjust to a world other than that of their siblings. You cannot be there to protect your children throughout their life.

I have a dear friend who had a wonderful son. She loved him dearly and always took good care of him and gave him everything he ever wanted. He was an only child and when he left home he had no idea how to deal with the world. Since he had never faced any real challenges or obstacles, to him the outside world was much crueller than he ever imagined. Be mindful in preparing your children for the outside world. They need to be aware that it may not live up to their expectations. It isn't always 'fair', it just is.

DISCIPLINING

Unlike with most children, certain disciplines do not work with intuitive children. It will not work if you have a whining, crying sound in your voice when you discipline them. Screaming and yelling doesn't work with these children either. They will tune you out or be deeply crushed. The tone of your voice will be your greatest ally in disciplining your New Age child, the calm, collected, assured tone that says, 'You will do this, and you will do it now.' This form of discipline will work with your these children about 92.3 per cent of the time.

When it comes to discipline, many of these children are very sensitive and don't quite understand exactly what is going on. Unacceptable behaviour when a child is small should be handled then and there by a short time-out. Spanking will not work with these children, so use discretion in your disciplinary tactics. At the same time, as with all children, the New Age child will take advantage if they feel they can get away with it.

A major key to parenting and raising a New Age child is to remember that you are important as a parent. When you have self-esteem and you love yourself, the child will treat you with respect and esteem. One of the worst things you can do is to let the child rule the household, and in many cases this happens. Sometimes when people wait until later in life to have children, they allow them to run everything that goes on in their home. When the entire household revolves around a child, the child is likely to become very unreasonable, self-centred and demanding, and can very easily get completely out of control.

As the New Age child matures it is very important that the parents remember that these children are very sensitive and can actually discern if both parents are in agreement. If the parents agree simply for the sake of the child, the child will know this and become very discontented.

Also, when deciding on a disciplinary action, ask the child what punishment they feel would be appropriate. In many instances they will come up with something far worse than you would ever think of or do. Although you would always choose to encourage your child to learn with words of approval and encouragement, there must be boundaries and a time when 'no' means 'no'. If there are no boundaries, a child will often push to your limit.

TEENAGE YEARS

From around the age of 12 to 15 is an extremely hormonal time for children. The brain is now shifting into a different mode. It is the onset of the mating ritual, as nature intended. Among many tribes in the African nations this is the age when people begin to mate. Because the impulses of sexual energy are so high, the child becomes very emotional. Because of the shift of hormones in the body, you will notice dramatic behavioural changes. This is a difficult time in the raising of children.

Since the brain is oriented to survival in the beginning, small children will cling to their mother with love and tenderness, but as they grow and develop and enter the hormonal state, things change. Their bodies are changing and developing, and they are becoming sexually aware. When the hormonal changes begin, the primitive instincts in the brain take over. This is a time in nature where the primal kicks in. The ties between mother and child change. There is a different interaction between child and parent. In some cases there is friendship and in other cases the teenager begins to pull back. Choosing to be with their friends instead of their parents is natural at this stage. They are pulling away from the natural bonding with parents and bonding more to others that share the same sexual energies.

As they continue to develop, their bodies releases pheromones. Pheromones attract the opposite sex. There was a time when the opposite sex was very unattractive to children and little girls definitely did not want little boys around, but suddenly the boys are noticing the girls and the girls don't seem to mind having them around. For both sexes, the body develops faster than the brain's logic capacity at this stage. Urges begin to affect them and surge throughout their bodies.

Because of the chemical changes in their brain, teenagers now begin to act almost on instinct. This is a time when you notice the change in them. They become very centred on themselves, and parents often begin to say things such as 'Don't you care what happens around here anymore?' and 'Isn't your family important to you anymore?' These conversations have been going on for centuries. And along with being totally self-absorbed, the teenagers suddenly become very interested in the sexual conduct and energies of people around them.

If the serotonin and noradrenaline levels in the body are unbalanced, they will exhibit manic depressant disorders. Deep depression (not wanting to go on with life) is one of the symptoms of imbalance in the serotonin and noradrenaline levels. Others are aggravation, anger and the inability to express emotion. You can adjust the serotonin and noradrenaline levels intuitively. Changing the diet may help as well.

Because of the emphasis our society puts upon a high protein/low carbohydrate diet, many important lipids are left out that are necessary to balance the different hormones in the brain. A good balanced diet is very important. But, as many parents will tell you, it is difficult to get a teenager to listen to your advice concerning their eating habits. At this stage of their brain's development, they have a tendency to think they know everything about everything. This is part of the actual development of the brain. The frontal lobe is not yet fully developed, however, so many of these children fail to realize the repercussions of their actions; they tend to act without thinking.

At this point the body is developing rapidly in so many different ways that it's hard for the child to remain balanced. Many parents come to me and tell me that their children seem lost. These parents don't know what they're doing, don't know what they're supposed to do and are unable to make decisions for their children, while the children themselves are simply incapable of behaving rationally. We sometimes forget that these children are a combination of young adult and child that is growing and developing. If we could just remember that it took us a long time to be able to figure things out, we would be more compassionate with this age.

This is the age when I caution parents to watch what their children are doing intuitively. Many children, especially New Age children, become remarkably intuitive at a very young age. They are able to see guardian angels and spirits. As they grow and gather more perception, they have many spiritual experiences.

One of the experiences they tend to have at a young age is that of making friends with entities or spirits, including wayward spirits. These spirits sometimes take hold of the children and tell them to do things that they shouldn't do. Because these children are very intuitive, they mistakenly think it is their intuition at work rather than spirits, and they think of it as giving them power. Thus the spirits mislead them and take their power. They sometimes live off the *light* of the children. Those children who invite these spirits into their space for 'more power' are allowing these spirits to take energy from them. Unable to realize this, they give their power away. This is why they sometimes join cults.

It is normal for children at this age to be interested in the old ways of religion and to be curious about many different beliefs. I have met parents who are frightened because their children are studying strange belief systems. It's not actually 'bad' to have some knowledge of these belief systems, but you do need to caution your children wisely and tell them not to give their power away, especially to negative spirits. The Creator is the true power. If your children do have occasion to visit spirits, they always need to check any answer they receive with the Creator of All That Is and then they will be safe.

You must guide these children to use their intuition wisely and then they will have fewer tendencies to give their power away so freely while they are still young. Many children are so open to the world that they are susceptible to becoming victims. It is vital that you programme your children to know that it's OK to stick up for themselves and it's OK to say 'no'. This coaching should have started early in life, but it's very important to emphasize this through the teenage years.

One of the most important things that parents can do for their children is to let them know that their sexual desires and urges are not wrong and that it is entirely normal to have them. But it is also very important that the parents express to them how serious sexual relationships are and that they are giving part of themselves when they indulge in a sexual relationship. You can only do so much to coach and guide these children; they will make their own decisions. It's wise for parents to realize this. That's just the way it is. But it's also OK for the parents to say 'no'. I have watched parents just let their children go in whatever direction until they are 14 or 15 years old. By then it's usually too late. This is just plain ridiculous!

Around this time there will come a day when children will realize they don't have to listen to everything their parents say, and that too is another stage in development. Some of these little spirits will then decide to go out on their own to do something. When this happens, it's very important that the parent does not feel like a failure. They are still responsible for this child and must not relinquish that right of responsibility. Children aren't considered legally responsible, at least in the United States, until they are 18 years old. But they will begin to make their own decisions before that. It's inevitable. The parent will just have to rely on the fact that the child was trained at a young age to have self-worth and is therefore capable of making good decisions.

Each child is special and each child's circumstances will be different. I have observed children using bad circumstances to the best advantage and I've seen children using good circumstances for their highest good. I am positive that the more you keep your children's minds occupied and active when they're young, the better your chances will be when they are older to influence them in the right direction. Get them involved in music or athletic training or anything where they can participate and stay occupied. This will help their brain develop and then they can go on in life using their abilities in different areas.

NINETEEN TO ADULTHOOD

When a child reaches 19 years of age they go through another development stage. This is when they sometimes assume that *now* they really are an adult. But they are not usually capable of seeing the outcome of their actions, because the frontal lobe is just barely developing. Girls' frontal lobes seem to develop a little faster than boys' as a whole, even in intuitive and New Age children. Allowing for the fact that each child is different, young men usually take a little longer to recognize the value of their decisions. They can hold a job much better a bit later, when they are in their twenties, and are more capable of raising a family then too.

Between the ages of 18 and 21 is the time when most children decide to move out on their own. Some may have tried this earlier, of course, and some may try it later. It is a big change to go into the outside world and take care of yourself. It can be a very frightening experience for a young person. As they move into adulthood they quickly learn that they don't know as much about the world as they thought they did. In some instances young people will try to set out into the world with a partner or mate, assuming it will be easier, but sometimes it is much harder to take care of a partner or mate. If they are prepared with the basics, such as the skills of maintaining a bank account, basic cookery and a few other things that are necessary to make it on their own, this stage of their life will not seem quite so difficult.

At one time manhood was not considered attained until the young man reached 32 years of age, because of the way the brain developed. This sounds pretty reasonable when you consider the 21 year old who comes home and tells you that he knows all there is to know about life and then starts offering you advice. This is amazing, isn't it, because if they really understood the world and life, they would race to move back home!

From the ages of 22 to 27 the young adults are becoming more and more aware of the complexities of the world. Somewhere between 27 and 32 years of age, they finally realize that they are just beginning to learn about life and become open and receptive to new avenues of thought. It is also at this age that they find their true mission in life. However, there are many New Age children who are aware of their true mission much earlier than this. Part of the reason for this is that they are rushed for time.

Bear in mind that many children born today are Children of the New Age. This information is given to assist you in making certain that your children are balanced physically, mentally and spiritually and that there is a balance in the body's hormones and in the brain so that the child is not manic depressive, angry or malicious.

The basic pattern of the New Age child is the fact that they have no prejudices. There is no prejudice against religion, colour, creed, race or anything that so often presents as prejudice to the world. These children are loving, kind and supportive. Because their brains are balanced with both male and female energy, they often have confusion about sexuality. They find themselves attracted to a person's energy rather than their sex and some of them bounce back and forth, assuming they are bi-sexual. Giving them good guidance will allow them to be who they truly are.

CHILDHOOD PROBLEMS AND CHILDHOOD DISEASES

ALCOHOL ABUSE

For most people one alcoholic drink isn't necessarily bad. There are some people who use alcohol but never abuse it. What is amazing is how fast alcohol can zip right into the mid-brain. In fact, it gives people a quick jolt of joy and satisfaction. For some people, however, alcohol can make them extremely miserable, especially young adults. The pleasure centre in the mid-brain, or 'reward system', is designed to ensure survival, not cravings. Pleasure is supposed to be a reward for sex, eating, success and other forms of behaviour necessary to survival. There are also emotional boosters such as satisfaction for a job well done. The brain is stingy about dealing out this pleasure. People wouldn't be motivated to work if their brain constantly gave them a supply of wonderful sensations.

It's very important that the pleasure centres of the brain do reward us, for when we are hungry, we eat. And if sexual behaviour were not rewarded by great pleasure, the human race wouldn't survive. We wouldn't want to have sex and wouldn't have children.

The pleasure centres release something called dopamine, which gives us a pleasurable sensation. It is very much linked to serotonin. Under normal circumstances, it works all the time, but when alcohol is added to it, it triggers the pleasure centres. Up until recently alcohol was thought to dissolve the brain tissue. It has this effect, but not the way we once thought it did. We now know it dissolves both water and fat, the two components of brain cells, forcing these cells to create emotions ranging from euphoria to depression or from calmness to aggression. We know that there is not one 'alcohol' gene, but there are some genetic disturbances in mutated genes that make people more prone to alcoholism. The tendency for alcoholism is definitely present when there is a low serotonin level in the body.

There are some good things alcohol does. If you're an occasional drinker, it can lower your cholesterol. Some amounts can prevent clogging of the arteries, prevent blood clots and actually ease menopause and reduce the risk of heart disease. If you drink just a small amount each day, it can stimulate your brain to function better. However, drinking to excess can cause great brain damage. It can cause the brain to start to shut down millions and millions of neurons. Russian men, for instance, drink the equivalent of three and a half bottles of vodka a week, and their life expectancy is about 55.

Being as inquisitive as they are, children will often experiment with alcohol and other drugs when their serotonin levels are very low. Because alcohol triggers the pleasure centres of the brain, they easily become addicted. Then alcohol starts to damage the brain, changing receptors and turning others on and causing a complete change in the personality of the child. Most parents don't want to watch their children change into something they don't understand. It's really important for them to step in and make sure that this isn't happening to their child, at least while they have control of that child. This is a hard decision to make, but young alcoholics are very dangerous, not only to themselves but also to others around them. Unable to think rationally, people will do irrational things to stimulate the pleasure centres.

When a teenager is young, the brain is very curious, experimenting and trying many different things. Good coaching can keep children on the right track. Lots of love can pull them back if they have pulled away. But it's very important that you let your children know at the very beginning that they have some self-worth, because alcohol and other drugs will destroy most of their self-worth over a short period of time. They will take what the children have spent years building and gradually diminish it into nothing, because they damage the receptors of the brain, and there's no telling what programmes they may keep and what programmes may suddenly be short-circuited. Reasoning and rationalizing will not always work when it comes to these young adults. Stepping in and being there to make sure addiction doesn't occur is the only way to keep it from happening.

Cocaine and other addictions can create behaviour that you would never believe your child was capable of. Too much drug use will also cause various changes in the brain. If you go in and start changing the neurons around and command the serotonin levels to change, however, it will create a difference in the need for that particular substance. Once the brain has learned that it can trigger these pleasures, it is very important that you teach it not to do so.

One thing that is important to understand about alcoholics is that so many receptors are being turned off and turned on with the use of alcohol that when alcohol is no longer used in that person's life, their serotonin levels will fluctuate a great deal. People who were alcoholics for many years will go back and act the way they were before they were alcoholics. So if they began drinking at 18 and quit when they were 40, their brain will go back to developing in some ways like that of an 18 year old, thus making the person a little immature until their brain can catch up with itself. This is why sometimes people who have great addictions and have recovered from them find life a little more difficult.

As a healer, go into the body to witness the serotonin and the dopamine levels returning to normal. Release the programme of 'I am addicted to alcohol' and replace it with what the Creator tells you. Ask the Creator what else to do; sometimes people need someone who is prepared to deal with their withdrawal.

You do need to prepare for some kind of withdrawal, because the receptors in the brain that were quieted down by the overuse of alcohol will suddenly be reawakened. There may be more receptors and neurotransmitters awake than before and it will take a while for the brain to readjust.

ASTHMA

When children have asthma, it is very important to realize that it is sometimes caused by emotional problems in their life. If a child has been taught to release more noradrenaline than normal, it will cause problems with the adrenals, affecting the likelihood of asthma developing. If a child is under a lot of stress, they may respond to it with asthma. But some cases of asthma are actually caused by fungus. If you clean the fungus out of a person's body, asthma can go away. It is a reaction to different allergies.

Asthma resulting from sensitivity to specific allergens is known as extrinsic. Causes of extrinsic asthma include pollen, small scales of animal skin, house dust, mould, feather pillows, food and any kind of solvent that contains something that the child or adult is sensitive to. Asthma affects more boys than girls, at least twice as many under the age of 10. Extrinsic asthma usually begins in childhood and can actually become dormant for a while before coming back in adulthood. Conditions such as fatigue and emotional stress can bring about an increase in asthma attacks.

Mild asthma causes infrequent wheezing and coughing. With moderate asthma there is a respiratory dysfunction and much more coughing and wheezing. Severe asthma is referred to as respiratory distress. The chest will make contractions and it's very difficult to breathe. Respiratory failure due to asthma is when there is almost no breath coming into the body. There can be impaired consciousness and the chest is silent, with no coughing. If this happens, the person can very easily die.

In mild asthma, there is usually no more than one attack per week. There is no sign of asthma between episodes and no sleep interruptions. In moderate asthma, the attacks can occur more than once a week. There is coughing and often there are more attacks at night. In severe asthma there are frequent and severe attacks, daily wheezing and very poor exercise tolerance. Inhalers have to be used the majority of the time; however, they do not reverse all the obstruction. Nevertheless, there are several medications on the market that are beneficial and can even make asthma somewhat controllable.

If you want to improve the asthma, there are certain things that can be done. One that is very helpful is to take the person off all processed flour and white sugar. This makes a huge difference almost immediately. Using myrtle, oregano and a product called Fungi Cleanse seems to help kill any fungus that is causing the asthma and clean out the body. With children, starting them on a good vitamin and one of the high-mineral group supplements also helps. You do need to be careful with vitamins and use them according to the child's age, etc., but vitamins and a good mineral supplement seem to make a huge difference. Drinking lots of water makes a significant difference also, as do blue-green algae and chlorophyll. Both blue-green algae and chlorophyll help stimulate the adrenals. Use the belief and feeling work to release programmes or add feelings as needed.

Some parents take their children to allergy specialists for injections to help with their asthma. This, too, is an effective method of treatment.

DHEA is helpful in some cases of acute asthma. However, some of the best results that we've witnessed have come from changing the diet and exercise. If the person with asthma has had a lot of stress and sorrow as a child, changing the beliefs 'Life is sad' or 'Life is sorrowful' or 'Life is hard' can help a great deal. In our society we have so many pollutants that actually attack the membrane of the lungs that being able to relocate to a place where the air is clean and pure would be ideal, but that is not always possible. However, removing flour and sugar from the diet, which can be done anywhere, seems to have a positive effect.

Never take an asthmatic off their medication – allow their doctor to make that decision – and never cause them to feel ashamed about using their medication. Until their body is ready and the fungus is cleaned out of it, their asthma will not improve.

AUTISM

Autism is a problem with the nervous system. It is a developmental disorder and usually manifests before the child is three years old. Signs of autism include self-absorption, lack of reaction to other people, sometimes banging the head against a wall. The evidence indicates that it is a nervous disorder. It can also be a genetic disorder, it can be caused by brain injury before or after birth and there's speculation that it could be caused by venereal disease or viral infections.

Four times as many boys suffer from autism than girls, and there are varying degrees of it. Children with mild autism can become very high achievers when they grow up. Children with more severe autism avoid physical contact and show no signs of understanding. Many of them do not attempt to communicate, but some of them will make gestures and sounds.

Medical science believes there is no cure for autism. Doctors believe that children with autism should be assessed by an experienced psychologist and placed in programmes that might help them. They have never discovered a medication that helps autism; however, we have found that going in and asking the Creator to put the child's spirit back into their space actually helps autism.

There are two kinds of autism that I see in children. The first kind is caused by a tragic birth or trauma during birth. It is as if the spirit is pulled a little bit away from the body during the process. These are the easiest of autistic children to fix. We find that the lack of communication and the inability to communicate can be changed by commanding the body to go back to foetal memory and to develop as a normal child. It *feels like* part of the spirit of the baby is trying to flee or came very close to leaving and isn't quite in its own space. Gently placing the spirit back into its own space will help.

The other form of autism that I've observed seems to be caused by too much mercury in the system. I believe this mercury is coming from vaccinations as well as though the mother's milk. And so no matter how many times you put the energy back into the body, the body will not hold that energy because mercury is being reintroduced into the system. Giving the child extra apple juice will help pull out the mercury and commanding the Creator to change the mercury may heal the child.

Never command any of the heavy metals to be completely pulled out of the body, however, because the body is made up of metals. If you command too much of the mercury to be pulled out at once it will make the body very ill, even if you replace the mercury with another energy that isn't mercury.

Where healings are concerned, the response from children who have autism has been extremely good. Making sure that the child feels constantly loved will break through the barrier which keeps them from communication, but pulling the heavy metals out is the key here.

BRAIN DAMAGE

Sometimes parents add to the difficulties of children who have problems with the brain. In some cases of cerebral palsy, where there has been a lack of oxygen at birth causing brain damage, the parents accept that the child is handicapped. If this is their attitude, the child *will* be handicapped. It is very important to constantly reassure a child like this that they are wonderful, beautiful and intelligent. Children who are encouraged by their parents to be intelligent and wise and told they are progressing all the time will actually start to progress. Children who are told they can do nothing will accept it as a programme and do nothing. I have watched this happen many times.

To work on children who have any kind of brain damage, you simply go into the brain and command the cells to become whatever they need to become. (If a child cannot give verbal consent, you must get verbal consent from the parents to work on the problem.) If the frontal lobe or the right side of the brain is damaged, ask God to show you the problem and command it to change. As you command it to heal, the foetal memory in the child's brain will start the repair immediately. If you are unfamiliar with different parts of the brain, all you have to do is ask the Creator to show you what needs to be done and witness it. Waking up a child's brain is easy. Teaching it what it is supposed to do is simple. All you have to do is command it to be so and let the stem cells and the brilliance of an infant's mind go to work.

Every time I work with children, I go up and ask their higher self if the condition they are in is the choice they have made or if they would like to change it. I always get an answer. If you're working with children who have been born with birth defects, it's also very important to do much of the work on the mother or the father (usually the mother) on the genetic levels. Anytime a child is born with genetic defects, you need to work on the mother's core beliefs. Find out what she believes and any genetic programmes that she is carrying. If you work on the mother, it will change the child.

If the child is born with Downs Syndrome, you simply witness God doing the healing. I have watched incredible changes happening with these children. One little boy had Downs Syndrome so badly that he couldn't do anything. But after the Creator had worked on him only once, he began to play with everything in the cupboards and communicate in such a way that his mother wept when I talked with her later on the phone. The Creator can heal anything and it's a false belief system that children born with birth defects are born that way because they did something wrong in a past life. I truly believe that you can carry many genetic programmes through your parents, but simply asking the Creator to repair them could change many of them. Granted, some of us want the experience of birth defects, but many would like the experience of living healthy lives.

A child must give verbal consent if there is any kind of genetic work to be done. If they can speak, they must tell you, 'Yes, I want to change this.' If they are too young to speak, but their higher self says, 'Yes, you can change it,' then you can.

Remember to constantly encourage children. When my youngest daughter was growing up, I used to look at her and say, 'Oh, you are so smart you could be a doctor.' And she would always say that she wanted to be a doctor. When she was 17 years old I said to her, 'Honey, think about this. Do you want to be a doctor or not?' She said she did, but I sometimes wonder if I simply programmed her to be a doctor. She easily gets As in school and is truly brilliant. She could be a doctor, but that's her choice. You should constantly be telling your children when they are growing up how wonderful they are. Allow them to make their own choices, within reason. Children fail when they believe they are going to fail; children succeed when they believe they can succeed.

The Creator showed me that we are only computer programs of what our DNA imprints. It is the life force that's inside us, the life force that is carried in the mitochondria of the cells, that is the very essence of our being. That life force can change anything in our DNA if it so chooses. That's right; our life force can make major decisions. We don't have to accept all of our handicaps. I hear magnificent stories of people who have accomplished great things in spite of their handicaps. They have learned how to paint pictures using their toes. Nothing stops them. People can change physical disabilities by commanding healing in the right and proper format, which is allowing the Creator to heal the disability, accepting the healing and watching it being done.

BURNS

Burns heal tremendously fast with small children. Going in and commanding their body to heal completely will do amazing things. When the child is first burned, command that all the pain be gone. It's the pain in the nerve endings that makes the burn worse. If you can dissolve the pain in the skin, you'll stop the burn from going in deeper. It will stop immediately and will cause no skin damage. In a severe burn, the nerve endings radiate total pain. This creates a shock wave that destroys more nerve endings, causing great destruction to the tissue. Command that all pain is relieved, the burn is completely gone and the body is completely healed.

Sometimes the shock of seeing a deep burn will send you into absolute panic, so be sure to put your hand over it or throw a towel over it (making sure it's clean and dry, especially if it's a deep burn) and command it be healed.

CANCER IN CHILDREN

There is an epidemic raging with our children and it's their susceptibility to cancer. Because of the different toxins and heavy metal poisoning in our environment, children are prime candidates for cancer. However, children with cancer, especially Children of the New Age, heal very quickly when given a healing.

When working with a child with cancer, it is important to also change their diet. In some cases of leukaemia, pulling out the heavy metals and radiation will change the body faster than anything else.

Cancerous brain tumours are very easy to work on. Don't let the idea of the child having cancer cause feelings of fear. Fear, doubt and disbelief can prevent the healing from taking place. Otherwise, children heal very quickly. When their brain is told what to do, it does it. It can go after and destroy a tumour rapidly. In many cases, large tumours begin to dissolve almost at once after a healing, and within a week they can have gone completely.

Do go up and ask the child's higher self if this is something they want to have done, though. Many of them will choose to be healed, but sometimes children will choose to leave this Earth, and that choice must be respected.

If the parents have sought medical help, always encourage them to continue with the treatment. As the doctors see the child heal, they will take notice, and the tests they are performing can be used for your benefit. With the use of X-rays, MRIs and CT scans doctors can detect shrinkage in the size of the tumours immediately. When they go in and see there is no brain tumour, for example, they will know the body is healed.

When parents come to me and ask if they should use alternative or conventional medical treatment, I explain to them that this is their decision and theirs alone. Never tell a parent that they should follow one plan or another. Alternative healing is very wonderful, but the medical profession is as well, and one day the two disciplines will work together in a co-operative way. In my experience people should make their own decisions about what to do. If they feel that chemotherapy is the right approach, then that is what they should do. Chemotherapy has worked very well on small children.

As a healer, you must abide by whatever the parents decide, difficult as that may be. I watched one mother let her child die of Hodgkin's disease, which is a treatable cancer. With treatment, it is likely that this child could have been given many years of health. But the mother decided that the child didn't want chemo, so they didn't do the chemo. The mother decided the child didn't need vitamins because she didn't like to take vitamins. Then she decided that the child didn't have to eat if she wasn't hungry, and the girl actually died of starvation, not Hodgkin's disease. Rather than seeking adequate medical care, the mother allowed her daughter to die.

This woman knew that her daughter was very ill. She also knew that she had terrible problems with her father, yet she forced her to be constantly in the presence of the person who was the cause of so much stress to her little body.

Under the right conditions, however, I am always amazed by how fast children heal. I have watched them heal instantly. A woman called from Argentina to talk to me about her 10-year-old son. I knew when she called me that it was costing most of her money to call from a phone booth, but she had such faith and determination! Her little boy had a massive bone tumour in his leg, but his mother told me that I could heal him. So I went up and I asked the Creator to heal her son. Then in my mind's eye I witnessed the Creator healing the bone and the tumour.

Afterwards, I received an e-mail from the woman:

Hell-o, Vianna,
Remember the woman from Argentina with the 10-year-old son with a bone tumour? You healed him. We wanted to attend your seminar, only the immigration did not allow us to stay. Would you come and train a group in Argentina? You will please tell us how much the seminar is per person and how many members are possible. We are waiting to schedule with you.
Love again,
Maria Krista

 With a tumour, go in and command it to be gone, see it dissipate and see the body return to normal. This allows the body to know the cancer doesn't need to be there.

Little children heal so much faster because of their perfect faith and because their body is still growing. Utilize this advantage when you are working on children with cancer. Always make the command: *'Creator, change this and show me.'* Make sure that you finish all aspects of the healing.

DEAFNESS

If children do not learn how to hear before they are 10 years old, the cells that teach the brain how to speak will be gone. If this is the case, the child will have a difficult time learning to speak.

When working with children with hearing disabilities, always go up and ask the Creator to correct the hearing and also to awaken the cells that teach the brain how to speak. When working with an adult, watch God take the cells to foetal memory and create the cells that learn to hear. In the foetus, the stem cells will become any cells that the brain needs.

Foetal cells are so intelligent that they will create only what the body needs. Doctors can take a foetal cell out of the heart of a child and a foetal cell out of a part of another organ and change them around and these cells will actually become the cells of the new organ. When the body is damaged in any way, foetal cells know the correct repair to make. This is why some children are able to grow back limbs that were lost – they don't know that they can't. There are many documented cases where children have actually grown back hands and arms in situations where they have lost them.

Sometimes the brain can be programmed according to what others around it expect it to do. A lady and her friend brought her nephew into me and told me that he was deaf, autistic and mentally damaged. They asked if I could help him. I went up and asked the Creator to show me how to heal this little boy's ears.

The Creator said, 'Vianna, the boy can hear.'

I actually had the audacity to argue with the Creator and said, 'No, you don't understand, he is deaf.'

With infinite patience the Creator said to me, 'Vianna, he can hear you.'

I said, 'Please, Creator, they tell me that he can't hear. They brought him to me to be healed.'

The Creator told me, 'Vianna, this child can hear just fine. Show them that he can hear!'

I then went in to take a look to see if he could hear. I saw that everything in his ears was working correctly. So I questioned the people who had brought him to me. He was a four-year-old child, he couldn't sit still and he kept making blurting noises of 'Uh, uh, ah, uh' while waving his hands furiously around and making gestures and motions with his arms.

I watched as the two women were trying to speak to him. They were trying to communicate with him in sign language, looking at him and showing him sign language as they talked. The child simply went on doing whatever he was doing.

I looked at these people and said to them, 'This child can hear you.'

'No, he can't, he can't hear us,' they replied. 'He was born deaf. Look at him, he's doing his own thing.'

I told them, 'He's doing his own thing, wiggling and making noises, because that's what four year olds do. I'm telling you, he *can* hear you.'

'No, he can't,' the aunt said.

Then I said, 'Yes, he can. Look!' I calmly and quietly spoke to the little boy, saying, 'Sweetheart, go and close the door.'

The little boy listened, got up immediately and closed the door.

They gasped, 'That's impossible! He can't hear what we say. He must have read your lips.'

I told them, 'Yes, he can. Quit telling him he can't!'

I turned him around so he couldn't watch my mouth, just in case he had read my lips, and told him to go and close the door again. He got up again and obeyed.

The two women were amazed at the 'wonderful miracle' I had performed, but this is what had happened: the child had truly been born without part of his hearing, but as he had grown the cells in his brain had replenished his hearing ability. Able to hear but told that he couldn't, he didn't pay attention to the people around him. This enabled him to do basically what he wanted. The funny motions he made with his hands weren't autism – he was trying to communicate with the people around him the way they were communicating with him, by speech and sign language. His gestures of communication had been totally misinterpreted. Not only could he hear completely, but he could also understand.

DEPRESSION

If a child is depressed, a good mineral and vitamin supplement may be needed. You can then command the serotonin to be balanced in the child's body. If the child has been inundated with heavy metal poisons, you need to give them a good mineral supplement to pull these heavy metals out of the body.

Mercury is one of the most toxic of minerals and can make children very depressed. Amalgam fillings should be taken out of their mouth and replaced with the ceramic type. The pectin in apple juice will pull out mercury from the body.

DIET

Another serious problem in our society is the diet of young people. There's very little real nourishment in a bag of crisps. The amount of chocolate and number of sweets that are consumed are outrageous. Removing white flour and white sugar from your children's diet might truly help their disposition. It might also make them outcasts among their peers!

Removing some things from their diet and adding wholesome food will help make them healthy and strong, but they need a good vitamin and mineral supplement as well.

INFLUENZA

Our bodies are created with the capability to fight off viruses. Do not command that viruses be destroyed in small children; rather command that their body fights the virus. This teaches the T-cells to fight viruses later in life.

There are some exceptions to this, such as hepatitis C. In these cases, ask the Creator to heal the child.

INJURIES

Once the brain has accepted the fact that the body is damaged, it complicates things. Once a healer sees the effect and the trauma of an actual burn, for example, their brain has accepted the burn. If they don't see the trauma, their brain hasn't accepted it, so they can command the skin to fold in perfectly and the brain accepts a perfect healing. This is why healings taking place inside the body are sometimes faster than healings taking place outside the body.

Children have so much faith that if you tell them something can be done, they believe it can be done. With that extra faith, their bodies heal 62.9 per cent faster than those of many adults, simply because they believe it can happen.

Children's bones heal so much faster than adults' because of the different growth hormones and because their beliefs don't block them. In repairing a child's bone, you command the bone to heal instantly by going to the Seventh Plane.

SPEECH PROBLEMS

Children who have problems understanding what other people are saying to them will have difficulty in being able to communicate and being able to read. Many children have speech and reading problems because their brains cannot distinguish consonant sounds. Consonant sounds are spoken much faster than vowels and as a result it is difficult for some children to distinguish sounds such as 'dah' and 'bah'. Normal children take 10 milliseconds to distinguish between two consonants. In children who are speech impaired, it takes hundreds of milliseconds to recognize the difference in the parts of speech.

It has been discovered that one way to help such children is to slow down the consonant sounds for them. Slowing down the language, reading very slowly, talking very slowly and playing back the words for the children teaches their brain how to distinguish the sounds. This helps speech problems.

STROKES

Young children can correct a stroke episode and become perfectly functioning adults simply because of stem cells. When working with any child who has suffered a stroke, go in and command the body to totally replenish itself and work with the stem cells. When working with an adult with a stroke, go in and ask the body to wake up the foetal memory to go in and change the things that are needed in the brain. Go in and say, 'Creator, show me.' This is the fastest way for the brain to reproduce itself.

In cases of stroke, the brain has too many dead cells. It must go back and re-create them and relearn. Sometimes relearning how to walk and how to move certain limbs takes some time, but overall, what we think of as some time is really not that long. It may take you a month to relearn how to move your arm, but it took you months when you were a baby. So be patient.

These are just a few of the conditions you'll work with. For more information, please seek classes on ThetaHealing's Intuitive Anatomy.

For more information on how to train your psychic child, seek ThetaHealing classes for Rainbow Children. The Rainbow Children course is designed to train the intuition of the intuitive child and adult.

LIGHT THERAPY

Children respond well to coloured light therapy. Our bodies can actually manufacture vitamins from various coloured lights, and healing can be greatly encouraged by the use of light therapy. You may choose to use this therapy in your endeavours to assist in the healing of others and yourself.

The following is a protocol that can be used for the treatment of illnesses and to promote good health.

Please note that when you are using light therapy in children up to the age of 12 years old, the treatments should be no longer than 30 minutes per session and the light should be applied from the navel upwards, encompassing the head, or on a single body part only, if that is the injured area. The lights should be positioned at a distance of 18 inches from the body. From the age of 12 years and beyond, the therapy can be used for up to one hour and used anywhere on the body as necessary.

THE PROTOCOL FOR LIGHT THERAPY

Anaemia and heart trouble: Green, lemon, yellow, magenta, red and violet

Asthma, hayfever and sinus problems: Turquoise, blue, green, lemon, magenta, orange and indigo

Cancer (leukaemia and tumours): Green, magenta, lemon and yellow

Cerebral palsy and other brain disorders: Indigo, magenta, turquoise, green and yellow

Colds and influenza: Green

Depression: Magenta, indigo and violet

32

THE FIRST SPIRITUAL INITIATION: JESUS THE CHRIST

Ever since I was a very young woman I have been having spiritual experiences. But my life was changed forever when I had a vision when I was 17 years old. I was married to my first husband, Harry, and pregnant for the first time. We had been married for nine months or so when Harry noticed that I had a difficult time reading. This was because of all the moving around that I had done up to that time. I would go to one school, only to be pulled out several months later to go to another, and this was not conducive to learning.

Harry stimulated my reading abilities in a crafty way. He would bring books home and read them to me. He would get me interested and then he would stop at a particularly good spot in the book and tell me: 'Now it is your turn to read the rest.' This would stress me out no end! But because I would be so intrigued by the book, I would start to read and comprehend better. The first book that he started with was *The Hobbit* by J. R. R. Tolkien. It was in this way that I started to take an interest in books. The next book that my husband brought home that stirred my interest was *The Lord of the Rings*. This was even more difficult for me, but it was such a good book that I got through it.

It was during this time that I was involved with organized religion. My mother had been involved with religion her whole life and was always talking about 'Jesus' this and 'Jesus' that. From an early age I could never figure this 'Jesus thing' out. I would think, 'Why would I pray to Jesus when I can talk to the Creator? Isn't that who we should be talking to?' I got myself into trouble with these statements when I was in church and when I was in my mother's presence. But at this period in my life things had changed in my young mind. I was married and I was going to be a mother. Now I became more involved in religion. I could still never understand the focus on Jesus, though, until my father-in-law gave me an old copy of *Jesus the Christ* by James E. Talmage.

By this time I had begun to read better, but this book was an even greater challenge. It fascinated me, though, with its insight into aspects of Jesus that I had never known. When I was three-quarters of the way through the book, I prayed to the Creator about the questions that I had about it. It was during the day and my husband was away at work and I nodded off to sleep with these burning questions in my mind. It was then that I had a dream that was so strong it was a vision.

In this vision, I was taken out into the cosmos to a faraway place where there was a beautiful beach. I intuitively knew that the beach symbolized the sands of time and the waters were the Sea of Knowledge. I saw a man sitting on a black rock that the incoming waves were breaking on. I knew that this was the man Himself, Jesus the Christ. He said, 'Hello, Vianna. We know one another.' After a slight pause, He added, 'You have questions about me and my life?' I said, 'Yes, Lord, I do.' Jesus waved his hand and said, 'Look!'

An opening into time was made and Jesus showed me all that was in his early life in the Holy Land. In a vision within the vision he showed me the truth of all the people that he had experienced in the time before the crucifixion. I saw the Sadducees and the Pharisees, the Romans and the Apostles. He showed me that he understood all of these people and bore none of them any ill will. He was the kindest person I'd ever met. He pulsated with a deep understanding of where everyone around Him had been coming from at that time and what was going on in the present. An incredible feeling of compassion came from Him. Then I asked Him about the end of the world and when it would come. What I saw was not what you would expect. I saw special children being born into the world. It was the birth of these children that would mark the end of the world as we knew it and it was these children themselves who were the new beginning.

I was so impressed and humbled by the incredible compassion that I felt coming from Him that I decided that if it was possible I would be as kind and compassionate as He was, or at least strive to be so.

I felt that I must give this incredible spirit a gift for the testament that was his life, for his compassion and mercy. I asked Him what I could give Him. He told me: 'Vianna, the greatest gift you can give me is to create something beautiful.' To Christ I gave the greatest gift I could give: the gift of my creativity. I made a vow to God and Christ that I would paint the 'End of the World' and 'The New Beginning'. Then I saw a vision of three murals that I would paint in the future. I also told the Christ that I would name the child that was in my womb in respect of Him. I named my son Joshua Lael. Joshua means 'Salvation of the Lord'; Lael means 'He is God's'.

Since that time I have studied many religions and have found knowledge in all of them. But I will always remember how I met the spiritual essence that was Jesus the Christ and the promise that I made.

I pray that you will listen to what the Creator tells you. I pray that you will know that the answers you receive are clear and real. I pray that you will be able to keep egoism out of the equation.

It is my sincere hope that you have found this book helpful to you in your everyday life and that you share this newfound knowledge with others. Most of all, may you come to know that between you and the Creator, no challenge is impossible.

EPILOGUE

Children of the New Age have great mastery from early on in life. As soon as they are able to speak, they sound as if they are old wise men trapped in a little person's body.

A good example of this is my own granddaughter, Jenaleighia. When she was three years old, her childminder, Connie, died. She had been my friend for several years. For many years we had depended on each other and had done many things for each other. I can easily say she was one of my closest friends and it gave my heart great peace and joy knowing that she was watching over one of my priceless grandchildren. I always knew she gave the best of care and kept my granddaughter safe.

When she passed on, my heart was deeply saddened, for I missed her very much. As I sat thinking of her one day, I remembered that she had collected crystals for years. Her crystals were her favourite possessions and she had placed them in many locations in her home. She looked after the children in her own home and they knew she loved her crystals.

I was sitting on the couch and my heart was so sad and I was missing my friend when Jenaleighia walked up to me, put her tiny hands in mine and, with her large brown trusting eyes looking into mine, said, 'Don't cry, Grandma. Connie is with God now, and God loves rocks.'

That little bit of inspiration reminded me of the joy my friend might be having at this moment enjoying being back with her Creator. My heart was filled with happiness at the thought. Jenaleighia's great gift of insight has often inspired me and filled me with awe, as things that seem complicated to me are so simple and easy to her.

It is our trusted responsibility as parents, grandparents, teachers, caregivers and health practitioners to nurture these magnificent and tender spirits with love and understanding. With the reading of this chapter, you will discover that many of you are Children of the New Age. You have a responsibility to teach others the way of love and compassion.

Appendix I

Quick Reference ThetaHealing Guide

READINGS

The steps of a reading are simple:

1. Centre and ground yourself.
2. Go up above yourself through your crown.
3. Go to the Seventh Plane of Existence
4. Connect to the Creator of All That Is.
5. Make the command.
6. Say, *'Thank you.'*
7. Say, *'It is done. It is done. It is done.'*
8. Witness with the Creator.
9. Rinse yourself off, ground yourself and make an energy break.

BELIEF WORK PRINCIPLES

Verbal Permission
We have the free will to keep any belief programmes we choose. Another person does not have the right to change our programmes without our verbal permission. Verbal permission is imperative to a person's free agency and personal integrity. So the person receiving the belief work must give full verbal permission to the practitioner to *remove and replace programmes*.

Also, the person receiving the belief work must give full verbal permission to the practitioner for *each and every individual programme*.

Witnessing
As with the readings and healings, the changing of beliefs must be witnessed.

Dual Beliefs
Many people have a dual belief system. For example, a person may believe that they are rich but at the same time believe they are poor. To correct this, leave the positive programme in place and pull the negative programme, replacing it with the correct positive one from the Creator.

Re-creating Programmes
Programmes can be re-created by the things we say, think and do. Positive action is needed to change our life.

Resolving Programmes
In the process of the belief work you may hear the Creator tell you that one of the other programmes besides the history level needs to be resolved, instead of cancelled, as would be the normal practice. Observe the energy being resolved on that level, as you would while working on the history level.

The Subconscious Mind
The subconscious mind does not understand words like 'don't', 'isn't', 'can't' and 'not'. You should tell the client to omit these words in their statements when in the belief work process.

For example, a client should not use a statement such as 'I don't love myself' or 'I can't love myself.' To properly test for a programme, the statement should be 'I love myself' and the client will energy test negatively or positively for this programme.

Working Alone or with a Practitioner
Some of the programmes that we carry have emotional attachments to them. So it may be rewarding to allow someone to assist you instead of removing programmes from yourself. Working with an experienced ThetaHealing practitioner is helpful, since the practitioner can find, assist and guide you in the proper replacement of programmes without emotional attachment.

However, some people are comfortable working on themselves. It all depends on the individual.

Pregnancy
Belief work should not be done with a pregnant woman in the first trimester to avoid liability. Belief work will not affect the foetus, but it is best for the practitioner to avoid these situations.

Negative Programmes
You can never command all negative programmes to leave the body because

the subconscious mind doesn't know which programmes are negative or positive.

Programmes within the Levels

A belief programme may be on any of the belief levels without being on any of the others. If a programme exists on more than one of the belief levels, it must be pulled and replaced from each and every level it is on for it to be completely removed. Programmes will re-create themselves if they are pulled on only one level and not on all of them. Explore the possibility that the programme is on more than one level. Pulling a programme from the soul level, which is the deepest level, will not necessarily remove it from the rest.

Intuitive Sensitivity

Intuitive people are more sensitive than others on all levels – mentally, physically and spiritually. In particular, they are very prone to being affected by low levels of toxic chemicals, toxic thought forms, spirits and Earth vibrations. Awareness of these sensitivities is important for everyday living, as well as for dealing with these energies. This over-sensitivity can be reprogrammed with belief work.

Words Have Power

Listen to what you say! The spoken word is incredibly powerful in a belief work session. If you find that a woman hates men, for example, do not programme her with 'I release all men', or she may leave her spouse and never be with another male. Pay attention to what you're programming a person with.

Use the Appropriate Language

Some core beliefs may have been created in a childhood language different from the one being used by you and the client. If this is the case, it is important that you both use the original language in the testing and command procedure. This is because the subconscious mind is so literal in its interpretation of information.

Early on in life, language becomes intimately integrated with mental concepts, thought patterns and memories. Even later in life, most people who speak a new language still think in their native language. The amazing part is that their thought patterns are still in sentence form. So, to get an accurate response with the muscle testing procedure, direct the person being tested to say the programme aloud in their native tongue (or in the language in which the programme was formed). As you say the commands with the

Creator, make the command that the programme be pulled and replaced in all languages. You can ask the client how to say the spoken programme in the correct language and use it as you would any other command process.

Ask the Creator
When teaching belief work, I am often asked, 'What do you replace the negative programme with?' My answer is always the same, 'Ask the Creator and witness the replacement as you are told.'

The practitioner is not allowed to change beliefs in their own way. The replacement beliefs should be divinely inspired.

For instance, when I am in a session I will energy test for various programmes. One of the most prevalent I test for is 'I am healthy'. You would be surprised at how many people truly believe they are not healthy. It might be necessary to release their current programme about health and replace it with 'I am healthy' on every level. Since each person is an individual, the replacement programme for health will be different for each person. I ask the Creator for the proper replacement programme to replace 'I am healthy, no'. I remove my ego from the healing and simply witness the beliefs released and replaced.

If you have any questions on replacing anything, you should always ask the Creator what needs to go in its place. Remember, the Creator will grant you anything if you keep your ego out of the equation.

EMOTIONS

Emotions are natural. Most of the time, they are for our benefit. Since we need our emotions, we do not attempt to pull *all that an emotion is* from a person. Fear, for example, gives us the incentive for fight or flight. It can also turn into anger, and a mother, say, may fight for her children. To take another example, we feel sorrow when a loved one dies. Grief should never be pulled from a person, as it is a separating process and necessary. There is a difference between emotions that are natural and those that are formed by us, voluntarily or involuntarily, and become obsessive-compulsive energy through our own force of will or the will of others.

Programmes, on the other hand, can be dysfunctional energy fields that, through the spoken word we create or accept as our own, are instilled in the brain or on the genetic/history/soul centres and cause repetitive or undesirable behaviour. However, when an emotion such as hatred is held onto for too long it can also become a programme that can cause problems to an individual. Good examples of this are the programmes of 'I hate my mother' or 'I hate my father'. It is permissible to pull and replace these since the emotion has become a programme.

A *feeling* can be an emotional response to love, sympathy or tenderness toward somebody. It is also 'the capacity to experience strong emotions'.

There are five different feelings that are our true feelings of emotion: *anger, love, sorrow, happiness* and *fear*. These are feelings that we experience every day of our lives. They actually save our lives. Although *anger* is usually thought of as a negative emotion, it is what drives a mother to protect her young. *Love* is the inexplicable emotion that cradles the world. The death of a loved one or friend causes deep *sorrow* within us. When everything is going right and we are content, we feel *happiness*. In a time of danger, *fear* will make us run, or stand and fight, depending upon the situation. All of these emotions at one time or another are necessary for our well-being. The mixture of all of them is actually an illusion of what we believe our feelings to be at any given moment.

These emotions can also be changed or altered by toxins and the chemical reactions of the body. Toxins and chemical reactions can both cause emotions such as depression. Not enough serotonin or not enough noradrenaline causes depression. Altering the DNA of the genes of the body can change these chemical reactions.

Emotions and feelings are what makes us truly magnificent and are a major part of our life experiences. All emotions, negative as well as positive, stimulate cell growth within our immune systems. It is when emotions such as anger and sorrow are allowed to grow unchecked and out of control that they have a negative impact on our bodies.

All of us at one time or another will have had a thought or feeling that we cannot get out of our head. A programme is a belief that endlessly loops in the mind, begging to be set free.

MINERALS

Since industrialized and big business farming was widely introduced, farmers have been using only three basic minerals for most ground crops: nitrogen, potassium and phosphorous. Each year that the earth receives this short shift of minerals, it becomes more depleted of the essential trace minerals we need to maintain health and prevent disease. In some places certain necessary minerals may no longer be found! No wonder many of the problems shown below, which are linked to the listed minerals, are so common:

Acne: Sulphur, zinc
Anaemia: Cobalt, copper, iron, selenium
Arthritis: Boron, calcium, copper, magnesium, potassium
Asthma: Manganese, potassium, zinc

Birth defects: Cobalt, copper, magnesium, manganese, selenium, zinc

Brittle nails: Iron, zinc

Cancer: Germanium, selenium

Candida: Chromium, selenium, zinc

Cardiovascular disease: Calcium, copper, magnesium, manganese, potassium, selenium

Chronic fatigue syndrome: Chromium, selenium, vanadium, zinc

Constipation: Iron, magnesium, potassium

Cramps: Calcium, sodium

Depression: Calcium, chromium, copper, iron, sodium, zinc

Diabetes: Chromium, vanadium, zinc

Digestive problems: Chlorine, chromium, zinc

Eczema: Zinc

Goitre (low thyroid): Copper, iodine

Greying hair: Copper

Hair loss: Copper, zinc

Hyperactivity: Chromium, lithium, magnesium, zinc

Hypoglycaemia (low blood sugar): Chromium, vanadium, zinc

Hypothermia: Magnesium

Immune system weakness: Chromium, selenium, zinc

Impotence: Calcium, chromium, manganese, selenium, zinc

Liver dysfunction: Chromium, cobalt, selenium, zinc

Memory loss: Manganese

Muscular dystrophy/weakness (also cystic fibrosis): Manganese, potassium, selenium

Nervousness: Magnesium

Oedema: Potassium

Osteoporosis: Boron, calcium, magnesium

Periodontitis (also gingivitis – receding gums): Boron, calcium, magnesium, potassium

PMS: Chromium, selenium, zinc

Sexual dysfunction: Manganese, selenium, zinc

Wrinkles and sagging (facial ageing): Copper

Please note: This is not a diagnostic chart, and it should not be used in place of your health professional to determine a recovery programme.

VITAMINS

All natural vitamins are organic food substances found only in living things, that is, plants and animals. With few exceptions, the body cannot manufacture or synthesize vitamins. They must be supplied in the diet or in dietary supplements.

Vitamins are essential to the normal functioning of our bodies. They are necessary for our growth, vitality and general well-being.

Vitamin Chart		
Vitamin A	Carrots, pumpkins, yams, tuna, cantaloupe, mangos, turnips, beet greens, butternut squash, spinach, fish, eggs	Poor night vision, macular degeneration, increased risk of cataracts, dry skin, hearing, taste, smell and nerve damage
Vitamin B1	Rice bran, pork, beef, ham, fresh peas, beans, bread, wheat germ, oranges, enriched pastas, cereals	**Mild:** appetite and weight loss, nausea, vomiting, fatigue, nervous system problems; **severe:** beri beri, muscle weakness, decreased DTR, edema, enlarged heart
Vitamin B2	Poultry, fish, fortified grains and cereals, broccoli, turnip greens, asparagus, spinach, yoghurt, milk, cheese	**Mild:** cracks and sores to corners of the mouth and tongue, red eyes, skin lesions, dizziness, hair loss, inability to sleep, sensitivity to light and poor digestion; **severe** (rare): anaemia, nerve disease
Vitamin B3	Chicken breast, tuna, veal, beef liver, fortified breads and cereals, brewer's yeast, broccoli, carrots, cheese, corn flour, dandelion greens, dates, eggs, fish, milk, peanuts, pork, potatoes, tomatoes	**Mild:** canker sores, diarrhoea, dizziness, fatigue, halitosis, headaches, indigestion, inability to sleep, loss of appetite, dermatitis; **severe:** pellagra
Vitamin B5	Whole grains, mushrooms, salmon, brewer's yeast, fresh vegetables, kidney, legumes, liver, pork, royal jelly, saltwater fish, torula yeast, whole rye and whole wheat flour	**Rare:** nausea, vomiting, fatigue, headaches, tingling in the hands, sleep disturbances, abdominal pain and cramps
Vitamin B6	Bananas, avocados, chicken, beef, brewer's yeast, eggs, brown rice, soy beans, whole wheat, peanuts, walnuts, oats, carrots, sunflower seeds	Anaemia, seizures, headaches, nausea, dry and flaky skin, sore tongue, cracks on mouth, vomiting
Vitamin B12	Clams, ham, cooked oysters, king crab, herring, salmon, tuna, lean beef, liver, blue cheese, camembert and gorgonzola cheese	Unsteady gait, chronic fatigue, constipation, depression, digestive disturbances, dizziness, drowsiness, liver enlargement, hallucinations, headaches, inflammation of the tongue, irritability, mood swings, nerve disorders, palpitations, pernicious anaemia, tinnitus, spinal cord degeneration
Vitamin C	Broccoli, cantaloupe, kiwi fruit, oranges, pineapple, peppers, pink grapefruit, strawberries, asparagus, avocados, collards, dandelion greens, kale, lemons, mangos, onions, radishes, watercress	**Mild:** poor wound healing, bleeding gums, easily bruised, nosebleeds, joint pain, lack of energy, susceptibility to infection; **severe:** scurvy
Vitamin D	Sun exposure, sardines, salmon, mushrooms, eggs, fortified milk, fortified cereals, herrings, liver, tuna, cod liver oil, margarine	**In infants:** irreversible bone deformities; **in children:** rickets, delayed tooth development, weak muscles, softened skull; **in adults:** osteomalacia, osteoporosis, hypocalcemia
Vitamin E	Vegetable and nut oils including soy bean, corn, safflower, spinach, whole grains, wheat germ, sunflower seeds	Rare symptoms may include anaemia and edema
Vitamin K	Green leafy vegetables including spinach, kale, cauliflower, broccoli	Rare, except in newborns, where bleeding tendencies are possible. Elevated levels of vitamin K can interfere with the effects of anti-coagulants
Zinc	Cooked oysters, beef, lamb, eggs, whole grains, nuts, yoghurt, fish, legumes, lima beans, liver, mushrooms, pecans, pumpkin and sunflower seed, sardines, soy beans, poultry	Change in taste and smell, nails can become thin and peel, acne, delayed sexual maturation, hair loss, elevated cholesterol, impaired night vision, impotence, growth retardation, increased susceptibility to infection

MERCURY POISONING

Percentage of 1,320 respondents indicating presence of symptom:

Unexplained irritability: *73.3%*
Constant or very frequent periods of depression: *72.0%*
Numbness and tingling in extremities: *67.3%*
Frequent urination during the night: *64.5%*
Unexplained chronic fatigue: *63.1%*
Cold hands and feet even in moderately warm weather: *62.6%*
Feeling bloated most of the time: *60.6%*
Difficulty remembering or using memory: *58.0%*
Sudden unexplained or unsolicited anger: *55.5%*
Constipation on a regular basis: *54.6%*
Difficulty in making even simple decisions: *54.2%*
Tremors or shakes of hands, feet, head: *52.3%*
Twitching of face and other muscles: *52.3%*
Frequent leg cramps: *49.1%*
Constant or frequent ringing or noise in ears: *47.8%*
Getting out of breath easily: *43.1%*
Frequent or recurring heartburn: *42.5%*
Excessive itching: *40.8%*
Unexplained rashes, skin irritation: *40.4%*
Constant or frequent metallic taste in mouth: *38.7%*
Feeling jumpy, jittery, nervous: *38.1%*
Constant death wish or suicidal intent: *37.3%*
Frequent insomnia: *36.4%*
Unexplained chest pain: *35.6%*
Constant or frequent pain in joints: *35.5%*
Tachycardia: *32.4%*
Unexplained fluid retention: *28.2%*
Burning sensation on tongue: *20.8%*
Headaches just after eating: *20.1%*
Frequent diarrhoea: *14.9%*

For more information in the United States, call 1-800-331-2303 Scientific Health.

Appendix II

Testimonials

Ken Best, Los Angeles:

I have witnessed a lot of unusual things in my life but nothing that prepared me for what I would experience in the world of Vianna's ThetaHealing.™

My very first experience was working with Vianna on a patient of mine who had seven brain tumours which were secondary to lung cancer. The woman was dying from the compression of the brain due to the tumours. I heard she was unconscious and unable to speak before going to hospital, basically in a coma after having a night filled with epileptic-type seizures due to the brain tumours.

Before leaving to go to the hospital I began working on her at a distance from home. Connecting to the Creator, I first saw her on the astral plane as lying in hospital with a sheet pulled over her head. Using ThetaHealing I took her astral body up to the Seventh Plane of Existence to bathe her in unconditional love.

When I arrived at the hospital she was unconscious. I continued to use ThetaHealing to heal her body and before I left she became conscious and talked briefly. By the next day she was lucid and talking. At this point she was able to have a phone consultation with Vianna. Vianna told her not to be surprised if the doctors couldn't find the tumours the next time they did a MRI brain scan.

I returned once more to continue ThetaHealing on this woman. Four days later the doctors stated that all the tumours, seen on MRI, had reduced by more than 40 per cent and determined that they were dying. At this point, after not being able to walk or move her limbs, the woman regained control of her body. It was truly amazing to witness.

My father was diagnosed with a deep invasive carcinoma of the oesophagus. This type of cancer has less than a 30 per cent survival rate even with surgery, radiation and chemotherapy. My father and I decided that there was no point to all the invasive treatments with little hope of a cure and the reduction of his standard of living if he went through all these treatments at the age of 79 with the removal of his oesophagus. He was also diagnosed with prostate cancer. I decided I wanted to have Vianna work with my father on the prostate cancer because of the possibility of some core belief issues that might be too personal for my father to discuss with me.

I was assisting Vianna, who was in Los Angeles teaching an Advanced ThetaHealing seminar, and during the seminar I was sitting in a very deep Theta state and decided to work on my father with a distance healing. I visualized entering his body after connecting first with God, and I saw the tumour inside his oesophagus. I asked God to show me what needed to be done to remove the cancer. I spoke with the cancer so it would realize that it was hurting my father's body and watched it disappear up to the God's light. The image was so strong when I arrived home I called my father and said, 'Don't be surprised if they can't find the cancer on the PET scan.' He went into hospital four days later to have the PET scan to determine the size of the cancer and they *couldn't find it*! He called me, very excited, saying they couldn't find the cancer!

Here's where the story gets really interesting. One week later the doctors called my father and said, 'Well, just because we can't find the cancer it doesn't mean you don't have cancer.' Then they said, 'You still have cancer.' As my father told me this I felt as though the cancer had come back, because his belief system ['Everything doctors say is true'] was so strong, as his generation believes doctors are infallible. At the time I said, 'Well now, I think you should go back in and have another endoscopic survey of the oesophagus.' Sure enough, they went in and found cancer. *However*, after a biopsy they found it wasn't the same cancer. The first cancer had been deep and invasive and this one was superficial, like skin cancer. It was easily treatable with a new photo-resonate therapy, which I suggested my father do because I felt he believed he needed a medical approach.

A year to the day later, the cancer came back in the same spot. At this point I had my father fly out from Florida so we could spend time clearing the emotional belief systems that were causing the cancer to come back. He went back to the hospital and they couldn't find the cancer. Hundreds of biopsies later, there's still no cancer!

Eric Brumett, New York:

I initially came to Vianna in need of physical healing. Since then my experiences with her as a practitioner and then as my teacher have led me through many healings, but I've gained much more than great health. I now have a whole new life full of love, joy, passion, prosperity, and so much more.

My first session with Vianna opened up my desire to have a clear awareness of life and all of its possibilities. I also became clear on my true passion, which was to help others do this as well. Vianna read this in me and invited me to her upcoming class. I immediately knew that I was going to attend.

Through this first and subsequent trainings I became a full-time practitioner and instructor of ThetaHealing, which has led me to a most wonderful and fulfilling life. The greatest change for me was that I was able to manifest, meet and marry my soul mate. We met through Vianna's classes and we now share our lives and a practice together.

As a full-time practitioner and instructor I get to share the wonderful benefits of ThetaHealing with people from all over the world. My students often go on to be instructors themselves and I feel honoured and touched to be part of what will be a legacy of healing that will grow and spread as it touches people around the globe.

The beauty of ThetaHealing is that it doesn't contradict other modalities; many of my students are practitioners of other healing arts and they are able to combine ThetaHealing with their own techniques for even better results. My students and clients are, in a word, amazed by their experiences with ThetaHealing because it works so well, it works so quickly and, most importantly, the results last! I can't imagine a more rewarding path for myself because my clients and students report remarkable results overcoming a wide variety of physical and psychological ailments. I get constant feedback and testimonials from my students and clients on how successful ThetaHealing has been for them. Every day I feel such love for Source and gratitude for all I have been able to create in my life. I am so very thankful to Vianna for showing me how to always connect with Source and for bringing ThetaHealing to all of us.

Bella Brumett, New York:

Vianna's own story of self-healing from a devastating condition which doctors predicted would end her life is compelling enough to draw many people to her seminars, but when you take her classes and learn her method of ThetaHealing you will yourself witness the most incredible changes in yourself and others. Although many people are drawn to this work for physical healing, the most amazing transformations are how much happier and healthier they become in all aspects of their lives.

By clearing our own issues of self-doubt, fear, lack of worthiness and any number of other self-limiting beliefs, we improve our own personal connection to our true selves and to Source. We are then able to do healings on ourselves and others that are beyond what most people imagine can happen but perhaps what they have hoped for all their lives. Being a student of Vianna's is a remarkable experience because you learn with an ease, joy and acceptance that is unprecedented. Also, unlike other modalities which may take years of study to even begin to use effectively, I was able to do ThetaHealing work right from the start.

I originally came to ThetaHealing because I was in need of healing for myself. Years ago, I was in constant pain due to injuries I sustained from being hit by a car while crossing a street. For two years I had sought relief and dared to hope for a 'cure' through conventional medicine, prescription medication, acupuncture and therapeutic massage. But relief from these modalities was only temporary and over time I was experiencing more severe symptoms, such as a loss of motor skills and reactions to medication. As is often the case when someone survives an accident where they narrowly escaped fatality, I was also questioning other personal and professional aspects of my life. And so it was that I asked the universe for an 'adventure', something new that would take me down the path of a more spiritual existence, not to mention bringing some much-needed joy and healing.

When I found Vianna as a teacher I was able to heal myself within mere weeks because ThetaHealing works in such a profound way More importantly, I was able to make the changes in my life that have led to a happiness that was previously elusive for me, including meeting and marrying my wonderful soul mate, with whom I now share a practice. Taking classes in ThetaHealing was a true awakening in my life; it makes sense, it's honest in its values and it works! Vianna is as humorous and loving as she is instructive. Taking classes with her has been joyful and enlightening and has inspired me to live with love every day through the practice of ThetaHealing.

If you wish to learn through unconditional love, humour (Vianna is an awesome story-teller) and compassion, instead of through fear and with difficulty, then ThetaHealing is right for you. If you wish to heal yourself and others in a way that is deep, meaningful and lasting, you will enjoy and embrace this method. The scope of ThetaHealing is difficult to put into words, but it brings the most incredible experience of being able to connect with All That Is and it will bring you understanding and healing on the deepest level.

Terry O'Connell, Idaho Falls, Idaho:

I first learned about ThetaHealing in late 2001. I found Vianna because I had been ill for seven years and no one knew what was wrong – not the doctors, not the homoeopath, not the Ayurvedic practitioner, not the herbalists, etc. When Vianna was able to pinpoint the source of this illness as long-term exposure to toxic mould, and to teach me how to do a healing on myself to change my cortisol level so I could breathe, she had my attention.

I hosted a workshop for Vianna in Los Angeles in 2002, where I became a certified ThetaHealing practitioner. Since then I have taken all of Vianna's workshops repeatedly and teach the work myself.

As a full-time professional ThetaHealing teacher and practitioner I have had the honour and privilege to witness many miracles. Early in my practice I witnessed partial blindness heal completely. I have seen cancer disappear, watched broken bones heal instantly, witnessed a second-degree radiation burn heal completely, seen hearing be completely restored to someone who was deaf without hearing aids, watched an eardrum perforated in a hit and run car accident heal, witnessed macular degeneration, cataracts and glaucoma disappear, watched SARS and West Nile virus disappear, watched migraines clear, witnessed Crohn's attacks stop within minutes, and witnessed thousands of physical and emotional healings. People unable to sleep for years have slept through the night after a single session. I've seen people become free of emotional scars that they have carried for over 50 years, including scars from internment in Nazi prison camps, abuse and the loss of a child. Many of these healings were proclaimed miracles by the doctors who confirmed them.

ThetaHealing has changed my own life in miraculous ways as well. I have recovered from the exposure to toxic mould which nearly killed me. My life is healthier, happier, richer and more abundant from applying ThetaHealing to my own issues. I have also been privileged to watch scores of students heal their bodies and their lives. ThetaHealing works, and it works miracles.

Katie Lamb, Idaho Falls, Idaho:

I have been fortunate enough to witness the wonderful work of Theta. Throughout the years I have witnessed personal changes in my life, as well as the lives as the people that I have worked with, ranging from people who have been healed from 'incurable' physical diseases to people meeting and enjoying soul mates.

My personal story of how instant Theta can be concerns myself and my youngest daughter, Rachel. There was an instance about eight years ago when a closet door at our apartment complex came off its hinges and began to fall in the direction of my daughter, so I went to push her out of the way. As I did, the door landed across my forearm as well as my daughter's forearm. Both of our arms were broken instantly … and healed instantly through the use of ThetaHealing.

I have also witnessed Theta healing autism. My granddaughter Aryn was the most beautiful child I had ever seen, but we began to notice when she was about 16 months of age that she began to withdraw from those of us who loved her and focus on one item for long periods of time. She refused to be held and would scream for hours while running in circles. This behaviour began to increase with age. I had seen and worked with people for a number of years doing Theta work, so we decided to work with my granddaughter. She began to accept the touch of love again and, instead of crying for hours on end, to carry on conversations. She knows that Theta works and that Theta heals.

This past summer (2006), Aryn was playing on her swing set like any normal four year old. She was hanging from the top bar by her knees when her mother came out to check on her and she dropped to the ground. A lump appeared on the back of her neck almost instantly, so we knew her neck was out of place. Her mother, my daughter Anna, had a cousin, my nephew, who had died from cancer when he was four years old, and it had started out as a lump on the back of his neck, so she was afraid that there might be something more wrong with her daughter. She decided to take Aryn to the doctor.

As Anna and the doctor conversed, little Aryn said to the doctor, 'Do you want to see how we take care of it?' The doctor said, 'Sure.' Little Aryn placed her hands on the back of her neck, leaned back on the exam table, said her prayer, sat up and the lump was gone.

Heidi LeMieux, California:

I have been blessed with the most wonderful gift ... having Vianna in my life! She has led me to develop my intuition and deepen my connection with God. After being healed by Vianna I proceeded to take *all* of her classes. Being able, through God, to heal others has changed my life. There is such a huge feeling of fulfilment in a way that is indescribable. I have never been happier or more satisfied.

Seeing people heal with Theta is amazing! My mother-in-law had hepatitis C, which she had got from a blood transfusion during open heart surgery. She suffered for many years before being diagnosed. Then she took the medicines available for hep. C. These only made her worse and she was forced to discontinue them. When Vianna came into my world she taught me how to work on hep. C. Miraculously, within a week my mother's symptoms had almost gone. She had pain and burning in her kidneys and liver, and these disappeared. Her liver enzymes were sky high and are now under control. Her fatigue, which had kept her in bed for days, is also gone. She now goes for vibrant daily walks with her granddaughter and is enjoying her life. Thank you, God; thank you, Vianna.

I have had the privilege of facilitating in many healings over the past five years. I have been guided in facilitating many healings of people who have been sexually molested as children and are for the first time able to move on with their lives. I have, with Theta, watched many with addictions be cured and those who were affected move forward successfully in their lives.

There is so much in detail I could tell, but I would need my own book. Let's leave the books to Vianna and let God bless her and guide her in our healings and our teachings.

Nini Gerard, Texas:

I have practised acupuncture for over 20 years and have been on the staff of Kaiser Hospital in California as well as on the staff of the Institute of Integrative Medicine. I have studied and worked with the most wonderful people.

I have believed for my entire life that there must be a way for all of us to learn to heal. I intuitively knew that reality was not as it appeared to be and that all of us were much more than we knew. All of us are born with gifts of healing. I know the ability to heal exists within all of us, just waiting to be discovered. I also know the gifts that I have are no greater than anyone else's. This I know to be true. Let me briefly share some of the things that I have witnessed since learning this technique from Vianna.

In 1999, a car hit my dog. Her back was broken in three places and her leg shattered. She had a pneumothorax and her heart was pushed to one side, she had internal bleeding and concussion. The vet said she had no chance of surviving the night. A year ago X-rays were taken of her. Dr Kaplan of Santa Rosa looked at them and to her astonishment, they showed no sign of any injury. The only evidence of my dog's accident now is the visible scars on her back.

In 2001, my mother was dying of renal failure and pneumonia. She was on oxygen and barely conscious. The doctors had abandoned all hope and let me take her home to die. In the morning, to the astonishment of all, she was sitting up eating breakfast outside in the sun and there was no evidence of any renal failure or pneumonia.

One of my clients, a young girl of 13, was terrified of dentists and also terrified of being put under or any other kind of anaesthesia. She had to have two teeth out and insisted that she do it without Novocaine and asked that I be present, so her mother and I went to the dentist's with her. A few minutes later, much to my astonishment, she emerged smiling! She had had her teeth out with no pain at all!

One day a client brought a man into my office who had given up. His body was riddled with cancer and there was nothing that the hospital could do. He had gone through radiation, surgery, etc. and they simply said that everything had been done. He and his wife were great believers and had heard about the technique. I placed my hands on him and asked that all the cancer be gone. I had a vision of him standing in the clouds saying he was fine and all was well. I took this to mean that he would be passing on very soon, and after he and his wife had left, I told my friend I was sure he would not last out the week. A few weeks later, to my astonishment, my assistant ran in to tell me there was a message for me that there was no evidence of cancer anywhere! I believe that his faith and the Creator's love healed him instantly, even though my own being had misinterpreted the message.

Once in San Francisco airport I was stranded without a phone and a dead battery. I had an old mobile phone that had not worked in months in the glove compartment. All I needed was for it to work once. It did and I was able to call for help. Afterwards it no longer worked, but I had been given what I needed!

I have had objects materialize and others transported to different places, and this has been witnessed. Again I must tell you the only truth I know is that we all are given these gifts and Vianna's technique will enrich your life in ways you can only dream of!

Sky Ahearn, North California:

A healing crisis led me to ThetaHealing and immediately I recognized it as the reason why I came to this Earth and knew that I had found my life's work. It answered questions that I had had all of my life. It helped me see how truly intuitive I was and I saw that it would allow me to do and be who I am without having to hide or be in a box anymore ... I could be the joyful person that I truly was, love people and help them realize the high potential that I could so easily see! I was thrilled and excited; my whole life suddenly made sense and seemed magnificently divinely orchestrated.

Ellen Cohen, New York:

ThetaHealing is an amazing energy-healing technique and process that is available and can be utilized by anyone, regardless of age, education, profession or other background. It transcends the 'typical' energy-healing techniques. It encompasses much more than a one-dimensional 'healing' technique. Instead, there are three main subject areas that come under the wide umbrella of ThetaHealing, and they are: (1) the healing techniques and exercises concerning physical, emotional and spiritual healing, (2) the belief work that changes negative beliefs to positive beliefs on four different levels, and (3) the fun and interesting metaphysical exercises. ThetaHealing is also a healing method of choice for practitioner, instructor and client, because with ThetaHealing, the Creator of All That Is is the healer and the practitioner is the facilitator. In addition, permission must have been obtained from the client or student prior to facilitating any ThetaHealing exercise that the Creator will perform. There must be actual knowledge and consent for every exercise conducted in ThetaHealing.

From my work as an Advanced ThetaHealing practitioner and instructor, I have witnessed many 'instant healings' and miracles conducted by the Creator of All That Is.

Concerning physical healing, clients and students have reported the following:

Release of pain (from neck, back, arms, shoulders, hands, face, head, stomach, etc.), and this release of pain continues after the session.

One woman reported that she had debilitating pain across her upper back, neck and shoulders. She had gone to several physicians and surgeons over the previous year, taken many medical tests, taken medication and reported that nothing had relieved her pain. Then, she attended a ThetaHealing experiential class that I taught and she said that during the class, after the Creator had conducted a couple of ThetaHealing exercises, she felt 'a tingling or electricity' going back and forth across the top portion of her back and then the pain had gone. Six months later, when I taught another ThetaHealing class at the same venue, she attended to report that the pain had never returned and she had been living pain-free ever since.

Use of extremities and full range of motion (i.e. instant healing on hand/arm).

Digestive disorders disappear after ThetaHealing.

One woman who attended a ThetaHealing experiential class that I had taught at a doctor's called me the next day to inform me that the 'spot on her lung' which she said had been evident on a test that the doctor had ordered for her had gone the day after she had attended the ThetaHealing class and experienced the various healing exercises done by the Creator.

After the Creator had performed a ThetaHealing and done four-level belief work, with a focus on resentment, on one woman, the bleeding and itching on her toes and feet stopped that day, and soon after she was rid of the fungus on her toes and feet.

Two students in a Basic ThetaHealing seminar that I taught reported that their vision improved 30 per cent after just the first day of the seminar.

Everyone uniformly reports that they feel tremendous peace after the Theta healings.

Concerning the four-level belief work, when clients and students experience the belief work, they and their lives are transformed. They are new people, with new positive beliefs and behaviour. I could write a book on the many transformations that I have seen, especially in the area of money, abundance, wealth and success:

People with no jobs or careers are suddenly, 'out of the blue', starting new successful careers with websites, businesses and clients.

Other people are growing their existing business with many new clients, new business contacts and connections.

FURTHER INFORMATION

THETAHEALING® SEMINARS

ThetaHealing is an energy-healing modality founded by Vianna Stibal, with certified instructors around the world. The seminars and books of ThetaHealing are designed as a therapeutic self-help guide to develop the ability of the mind to heal. ThetaHealing includes the following seminars and books:

ThetaHealing® seminars taught by certified ThetaHealing® instructors:

> ThetaHealing Basic DNA 1 and 2 Practitioner Seminar
>
> ThetaHealing Advanced DNA 2½ Practitioner Seminar
>
> ThetaHealing Manifesting and Abundance Practitioner Seminar
>
> ThetaHealing Intuitive Anatomy Practitioner Seminar
>
> ThetaHealing Rainbow Children Practitioner Seminar
>
> ThetaHealing Disease and Disorders Practitioner Seminar
>
> ThetaHealing World Relations Practitioner Seminar
>
> ThetaHealing DNA 3 Practitioner Seminar
>
> ThetaHealing Animal Practitioner Seminar
>
> ThetaHealing Dig Deeper Practitioner Seminar
>
> ThetaHealing Plant Practitioner Seminar
>
> ThetaHealing SoulMate Practitioner Seminar
>
> ThetaHealing Rhythm Practitioner Seminar
>
> ThetaHealing Planes of Existence Practitioner Seminar

**Certification seminars taught exclusively by Vianna at the ThetaHealing®
Institute of Knowledge:**

> ThetaHealing Basic DNA 1 and 2 Instructors' Seminar
>
> ThetaHealing Advanced DNA 2½ Instructors' Seminar
>
> ThetaHealing Manifesting and Abundance Instructors' Seminar
>
> ThetaHealing Intuitive Anatomy Instructors' Seminar
>
> ThetaHealing Rainbow Children Instructors' Seminar
>
> ThetaHealing Disease and Disorders Instructors' Seminar
>
> ThetaHealing World Relations Instructors' Seminar
>
> ThetaHealing DNA 3 Instructors' Seminar
>
> ThetaHealing Animal Instructors' Seminar
>
> ThetaHealing Dig Deeper Instructors' Seminar
>
> ThetaHealing Plant Instructors' Seminar
>
> ThetaHealing SoulMate Instructors' Seminar
>
> ThetaHealing Rhythm Instructors' Seminar
>
> ThetaHealing Planes of Existence Instructors' Seminar

ThetaHealing is always growing and expanding, and new courses are added
often.

Books:

> *ThetaHealing®* (Hay House, 2006, 2010)
>
> *Advanced ThetaHealing®* (Hay House, 2011)
>
> *ThetaHealing® Diseases and Disorders* (Hay House, 2012)
>
> *On the Wings of Prayer* (Hay House, 2012)
>
> *ThetaHealing® Rhythm for Finding Your Perfect Weight* (Hay House, 2013)

ABOUT THE AUTHOR

Vianna Stibal is a grandmother, artist and writer. After being taught how to connect with the Creator to co-create and facilitate the unique process called ThetaHealing, she knew that she must share this gift with as many people as she could. It was this love and appreciation for the Creator and humankind that allowed her to develop the ability to see clearly into the human body and witness many cases of instantaneous healing.

Her encyclopaedic knowledge of the body's systems and deep understanding of the human psyche, based on her own experience as well as the insight given to her by the Creator, makes Vianna the perfect practitioner of this amazing technique. She has successfully worked with such medical challenges as hepatitis C, Epstein-Barr virus, AIDS, herpes, tumours, various types of cancer and many other conditions, diseases and genetic defects.

Vianna knows that the ThetaHealing technique is teachable, but beyond that she knows that it *needs* to be taught. She conducts seminars all over the world to teach people of all races, beliefs and religions. She has trained teachers and practitioners who are working in 14 countries, but her work will not stop there! Vianna is committed to spreading this healing paradigm throughout the world.-

NOTES

NOTES

Hay House Titles of Related Interest

The 8th Chakra,
by Jude Currivan, PhD

Ask and It Is Given,
by Esther and Jerry Hicks

The Biology of Belief,
by Bruce Lipton

Emotional Balance,
by Dr Roy Martina

Instant Cosmic Ordering,
by Barbel Mohr

Matrix Reimprinting Using EFT,
by Karl Dawson and Sasha Allenby

Quantum Field Healing (CD),
by David R. Hamilton, PhD

HAY HOUSE

Look within

Join the conversation about latest products,
events, exclusive offers and more.

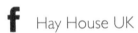 Hay House UK

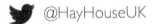 @HayHouseUK

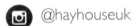 @hayhouseuk

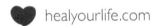 healyourlife.com

We'd love to hear from you!